296
Current Topics in Microbiology and Immunology

Editors

R. W. Compans, Atlanta/Georgia
M. D. Cooper, Birmingham/Alabama
T. Honjo, Kyoto · H. Koprowski, Philadelphia/Pennsylvania
F. Melchers, Basel · M. B. A. Oldstone, La Jolla/California
S. Olsnes, Oslo · M. Potter, Bethesda/Maryland
P. K. Vogt, La Jolla/California · H. Wagner, Munich

M.B.A. Oldstone (Ed.)

Molecular Mimicry: Infection-Inducing Autoimmune Disease

With 28 Figures and 9 Tables

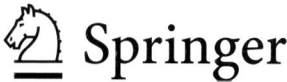

Michael B.A. Oldstone, M.D.
The Scripps Research Institute
Department of Neuropharmacology
10550 N. Torrey Pines Road
La Jolla, CA 92037
USA
e-mail: mbaobo@scripps.edu

Cover illustration by Melissa Nicholson and Kai W. Wucherpfenning
The cover shows the crystal structure of the first human autoimmune T cell receptor bound to its self-peptide/MHC target. The T cell receptor originated from a patient with relapsing-remitting multiple sclerosis and is specific for a myelin basic protein peptide bound to HLA-DR2 (DRA, DRB1*1501). This structure showed a highly unusual binding topology in which the T cell receptor only contacted the N-terminal part of the self-peptide. This binding mode reduces the interaction surface with the MHC bound peptide, and places physical limits on the peptide specificity of this T cell receptor. This structure thus provides an explanation for the finding that this myelin basic protein specific T cell clone can be activated by a number of different microbial peptides that have limited sequence similarity with the self-peptide. The MHC molecule is colored blue, and the TCR alpha and beta chains yellow and red, respectively. The peptide is shown as a stick and ball model.

Library of Congress Catalog Number 72-152360

ISSN 0070-217X
ISBN-10 3-540-25597-4 Springer Berlin Heidelberg New York
ISBN-13 978-3-540-25597-0 Springer Berlin Heidelberg New York

This work is subject to copyright. All rights reserved, whether the whole or part of the material is concerned, specifically the rights of translation, reprinting, reuse of illustrations, recitation, broadcasting, reproduction on microfilm or in any other way, and storage in data banks. Duplication of this publication or parts thereof is permitted only under the provisions of the German Copyright Law of September, 9, 1965, in its current version, and permission for use must always be obtained from Springer-Verlag. Violations are liable for prosecution under the German Copyright Law.

Springer is a part of Springer Science+Business Media
springeronline.com
© Springer-Verlag Berlin Heidelberg 2005
Printed in Germany

The use of general descriptive names, registered names, trademarks, etc. in this publication does not imply, even in the absence of a specific statement, that such names are exempt from the relevant protective laws and regulations and therefore free for general use.
Product liability: The publisher cannot guarantee the accuracy of any information about dosage and application contained in this book. In every individual case the user must check such information by consulting the relevant literature.

Editor: Simon Rallison, Heidelberg
Desk editor: Anne Clauss, Heidelberg
Production editor: Nadja Kroke, Leipzig
Cover design: design & production GmbH, Heidelberg
Typesetting: LE-TEX Jelonek, Schmidt & Vöckler GbR, Leipzig
Printed on acid-free paper   SPIN 11376323   27/3150/YL – 5 4 3 2 1 0

List of Contents

Molecular Mimicry, Microbial Infection, and Autoimmune Disease:
Evolution of the Concept 1
   M. B. A. Oldstone

The Structural Interactions Between T Cell Receptors
and MHC–Peptide Complexes Place Physical Limits
on Self–Nonself Discrimination 19
   K. W. Wucherpfennig

A Virus-Induced Molecular Mimicry Model of Multiple Sclerosis 39
   J. K. Olson, A. M. Ercolini, and S. D. Miller

Suppression of Autoimmunity via Microbial Mimics
of Altered Peptide Ligands 55
   L. Steinman, P. J. Utz, and W. H. Robinson

Molecular and Cellular Mechanisms, Pathogenesis, and Treatment
of Insulin-Dependent Diabetes Obtained Through Study
of a Transgenic Model of Molecular Mimicry 65
   M. B. A. Oldstone

Trypanosoma cruzi-Induced Molecular Mimicry and Chagas' Disease 89
   N. Gironès, H. Cuervo, and M. Fresno

HTLV-1 Induced Molecular Mimicry in Neurological Disease 125
   S. M. Lee, Y. Morcos, H. Jang, J. M. Stuart, and M. C. Levin

Molecular Mimicry: Anti-DNA Antibodies Bind Microbial
and Nonnucleic Acid Self-Antigens 137
   J. S. Rice, C. Kowal, B. T. Volpe, L. A. DeGiorgio, and B. Diamond

Chlamydia and Antigenic Mimicry 153
   K. Bachmaier and J. M. Penninger

Subject Index 165

List of Contributors

(Addresses stated at the beginning of respective chapters)

Bachmaier, K.   153

Cuervo, H.   89

DeGiorgio, L. A.   137
Diamond, B.   137

Ercolini, A. M.   39

Fresno, M.   89

Gironès, N.   89

Jang, H.   125

Kowal, C.   137

Lee, S. M.   125
Levin, M. C.   125

Miller, S. D.   39
Morcos, Y.   125

Oldstone, M. B. A.   1, 65
Olson, J. K.   39

Penninger, J. M.   153

Rice, J. S.   137
Robinson, W. H.   55

Steinman, L.   55
Stuart, J. M.   125

Utz, P. J.   55

Volpe, B. T.   137

Wucherpfennig, K. W.   19

Molecular Mimicry, Microbial Infection, and Autoimmune Disease: Evolution of the Concept

M. B. A. Oldstone (✉)

Division of Virology, Departments of Neuropharmacology and Infectology, The Scripps Research Institute, 10550 N. Torrey Pines Road, La Jolla, CA 92037, USA
mbaobo@scripps.edu

1	Definition of Molecular Mimicry and Development of the Concept	2
2	Occurrence of Molecular Mimicry at the Antibody and T Cell Level	4
3	Searches for Molecular Mimics	5
4	Experimental Animal Models of Molecular Mimicry and Autoimmune Disease	5
5	Equating Human Autoimmune Disease with Molecular Mimicry	10
6	Overview of Autoimmune Responses and Infections	11
7	Summary	13
	References	14

Abstract Molecular mimicry is defined as similar structures shared by molecules from dissimilar genes or by their protein products. Either several linear amino acids or their conformational fit may be shared, even though their origins are separate. Hence, during a viral or microbe infection, if that organism shares cross-reactive epitopes for B or T cells with the host, then the response to the infecting agent will also attack the host, causing autoimmune disease. A variation on this theme is when a second, third, or repeated infection(s) shares cross-reactive B or T cell epitopes with the first (initiating) virus but not necessarily the host. In this instance, the secondary infectious agents increase the number of antiviral/antihost effector antibodies or T cells that potentiate or precipitate the autoimmune assault. The formation of this concept initially via study of monoclonal antibody or clone T cell cross-recognition in vitro through its evolution to in vivo animal models and to selected human diseases is explored in this mini-review.

1
Definition of Molecular Mimicry and Development of the Concept

We initially defined molecular mimicry as similar structures shared by molecules from dissimilar genes or by their protein products (Fujinami et al. 1983; Oldstone 1987; reviewed in Oldstone 1998). Either the molecules' linear amino acid sequences or their conformational fit (Fig. 1) may be shared, even though their origins are separate. Examples would be self-determinants from a virus and a normal host or from two kinds of viruses, one that persists in a selected tissue with little or no injury until the second virus infects the same host and generates an immune response that cross-reacts with tissue expressing peptides from the first virus.

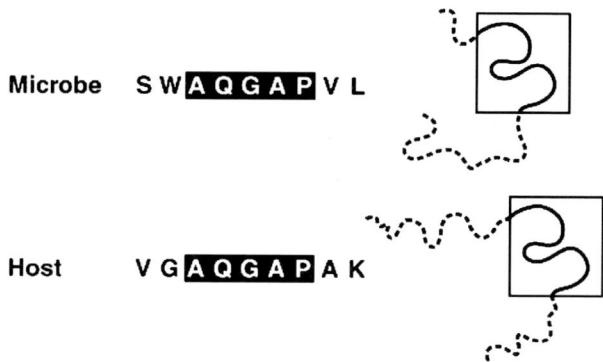

- Close enough in homology (between self and microbe) to share determinants.
- Distant enough from homology to be recognized as foreign by the immune system.
- Homology at self determinants (epitope) having important biologic activity.

Fig. 1 Cartoon of a shared linear amino acid sequence or of a conformational fit between a microbe and a host "self" determinant. This is the basis for the first phase of molecular mimicry. Autoimmunity can occur if: (1) a host immune response raised against the sequence from the microbe cross-reacts with the host "self" sequence, and (2) the host sequence is a biologically important domain, e.g., encephalitogenic site of myelin basic protein, the site on the acetylcholine receptor that is important for gating membrane changes needed for a synapse. A similar scenario might occur when, early in life, a virus or microbe initiates a persistent infection in a specific tissue, and a second cross-reactive infectious agent later induces an antiviral or antimicrobial immune response

The sequence homology between the infected host's self-components and those of the microbe must be close enough to share immunogenic determinants, yet sufficiently distant to be recognized as nonself by the host's immune system. Further, such homology must involve a self-determinant having important biological activity so that the immune assault injures tissue and causes disease (Fig. 1). For instance, we know that immune attack on the encephalitogenic peptide of myelin can injure oligodendrocytes and that similar violence to islet or myocardial surface-expressed peptides harms the pancreas or heart, respectively. Such homologies between proteins have been detected either by use of immunologic agents, humoral or cellular, that cross-react with two protein structures (virus–host, virus–virus) or by computer searches to match proteins described in storage banks. Because guanine-cytosine (GC) sequences and introns designed to be spliced away may provide false hybridization signals and nonsense homologies, respectively, focus on molecular mimicry is necessary at the protein level. Regardless of the methods used for identification, it is now abundantly clear that molecular mimicry occurs between proteins encoded by numerous microbes and host self-proteins and is rather common [reviewed in Cunningham and Fujinami 2000; Oldstone 1989, 1998; with over 500 published papers on this subject listed in PubMed from 2003 to the present (October 2004)]. This information is useful not only for research in autoimmunity but also to those seeking a likely mechanism by which viral proteins are processed inside cells (Dales et al. 1983a, 1983b; Oldstone 1998).

The conceptual basis for molecular mimicry was first defined in the early 1980s when monoclonal antibodies against viruses were also shown to react with nonviral host protein; in this case, measles virus phosphoprotein cross-reacted with host cell cytokeratin (Fujinami et al. 1983), herpes simplex virus type 1 with host cell vimentin (Fujinami et al. 1983) and vaccinia virus with host cell intermediate filaments (Dales et al. 1983b). After this discovery, others emerged, again at the clonal level, that T cell clones against proteins from a variety of infectious agents also reacted with host antigenic determinants (Cunningham 2004; Wucherpfennig and Strominger 1995). The clonal distinction was imperative for the initial definition of mimicry. At least 30 years before our initial description of molecular mimicry involving cross-reactions between numerous microbes, on the polyclonal antibody level, streptococcus was believed to react with renal glomeruli, heart ,and basal ganglia to account for glomerulonephritis, heart and valvular disease, and chorea, respectively (reviewed in Froude et al. 1989; Kaplan 1963). However, subsequent research showed that the nephritis was caused by immune complex deposits and the tissue damage they produced (Dixon 1963). Later, in 1990, the cross-reactivity of streptococcal antigen with myocardial antigens on a clonal level was uncovered (Dell et al. 1991). Hence, for both historical reasons and mechanistic understanding, it is best to provide evidence for cross-reactivity at the clonal level to prove that molecular mimicry exists.

2
Occurrence of Molecular Mimicry at the Antibody and T Cell Level

Critical analysis has revealed that molecular mimicry during the infectious process is not rare. For example, multiple monoclonal antibodies against a battery of DNA and RNA viruses were noted to be cross-reactive with host determinants (reviewed in Oldstone et al. 1998). Frequency of cross-reactivity between viral proteins and host self-antigens analyzed with more than 800 monoclonal antibodies revealed that nearly 5% of the monoclonal antibodies against 15 different viruses cross-reacted with host cell determinants expressed on or in uninfected tissues (Lane and Hoeffler 1980; Oldstone 1998; Shrinivasappa et al. 1986). The viruses studied were among the most common that afflict humans, including those of the herpesvirus group, vaccinia virus, myxoviruses, paramyxoviruses, arenaviruses, flaviviruses, alphaviruses, rhabdoviruses, coronaviruses, and human retroviruses. Considering that five to six amino acids are needed to induce a monoclonal antibody response, the probability that 20 amino acids will occur in six identical residues between two proteins is 20^6 or 1 in 128,000,000. Similarly, a variety of T lymphocytes sensitized to cellular proteins such as myelin basic protein, proteolipid protein of myelin, and glutamic decarboxylase (GAD) were also noted to cross-react when added to proteins or peptides from selected viruses. Biological/chemical analyses used to document these effects were amino acid sequencing, immunochemistry, cell proliferation, lysis, and the release or display of cytokines (reviewed in Cunningham and Fujinami 2000; reviewed in Oldstone 1989, 1998; Wucherpfennig and Strominger 1995). The reverse was also noted, in that T lymphocytes sensitized specifically to a virus would cross-react with a host protein or peptide (Oldstone et al. 1999). The permissivity of the T cell receptor to numerous peptides (Mason 1998) indicated that the problem was not the probability of multiple recognition but rather how the host limited/controlled such cross-recognition.

Computer searches revealed interesting sequence homologies that might explain a variety of diseases; for example, the amino acids shared between specific coagulation proteins and dengue virus or between human immunodeficiency virus and brain proteins could indicate part of the pathogenic mechanism underlying dengue hemorrhagic shock syndrome and AIDS dementia complex, respectively. Clinical studies have shown a high degree of correlation between the immune response to GAD and other islet antigens in patients who progress to or who have insulin-dependent diabetes. Sequences obtained by computer search revealed identity between a component of GAD amino acids 247 to 279 and other auto-antigens with several viruses (Atkinson et al. 1994; Honeyman et al. 1998). Similarly, evidence has linked chlamydia protein with heart disease, herpes simplex virus with corneal antigens, herpes viruses with myasthenia gravis (Bachmaier et al. 1999; Schwimmbeck et al. 1989; Zhao et al. 1997), the bacteria *Campylobacter jejuni* with Guillain-Barré disease (Hafer-Macko et al. 1996; Yuki et al. 2004) and certain strains of *Yersinia*, *Shigella*, and *Klebsiella* with ankylosing spondylitis (AS) (Oldstone 1998; Schwimmbeck et al. 1987). In these instances, the protein and antigen of the microbe acting as mimics and inducers of antibodies and/or T lymphocytes were implicated as likely causes of the respective diseases.

3
Searches for Molecular Mimics

As experimental knowledge increased about the T cell epitopes and their flanking sequences that were necessary for T cell recognition, it became possible to change a single amino acid and, thereby, convert a poorly binding T cell epitope to one that bound with high affinity and, vice versa, convert a strongly binding peptide to one of mediocre affinity (Table 1). Armed with this information, better designs for computer searches are now possible to identify molecular mimics. These data, coupled with interesting sequence similarities to evaluate, provide a list of microbial and host proteins worthy of investigation (Table 2). However, immunochemical analysis of cross-reactive epitopes has revealed that reactivity can be dependent on a single amino acid (Dyrberg and Oldstone 1986; Dyrberg et al. 1990; Hudrisier et al. 2001) (Table 1), so experimental evidence is required to support computerized identification of a sequence fit.

4
Experimental Animal Models of Molecular Mimicry and Autoimmune Disease

An essential step in validation of the molecular mimicry concept was obtaining proof of principle from animal models to establish molecular mimicry as more than an epiphenomenon. The initial observation utilized myelin basic protein and the model of experimental autoimmune encephalomyelitis (EAE)

Table 1 Effect of mutation at non-anchor position P2 on the H-2D^b binding properties of H-2D^b-restricted viral peptides

Peptide	Binding affinity Competition (IC$_{50}$, nM)	Stabilization (SC$_{50}$, nM)
Influenza		
NP366–374	7 ± 1	10 ± 1
Ala Ser Asn Glu Asn Met Glu Thr Met		
[Glu]^2-NP366–374	1,939 ± 109	12,350 ± 350
Ala Glu Asn Glu Asn Met Glu Thr Met		
LCMV		
GP33–41	21 ± 4	470 ± 63
Lys Ala Val Tyr Asn Phe Ala Thr Cys Gly Ile		
[Glu]^2-GP33–41	13000 ± 3790	53000 ± 8460
Lys Glu Val Tyr Asn Phe Ala Thr Cys Gly Ile		
GP276–286	13 ± 2	23 ± 3
Ser Gly Val Glu Asn Pro Gly Gly Tyr Cys Leu		
[Glu]^2-GP276–286	15067 ± 5715	43000 ± 5650
Ser Glu Val Glu Asn Pro Gly Gly Tyr Cys Leu		
LCMV		
GP16–24	>100000	>100000
Asp Glu Val Ile Asn Ile Val Ile Ile		
[Ser]^2-GP16–24	1400 ± 450	2050 ± 390
Asp Ser Val Ile Asn Ile Val Ile Ile		
[Gly]^2-GP16–24	2033 ± 887	4930 ± 721
Asp Gly Val Ile Asn Ile Val Ile Ile		

Substitution of a single amino acid can reverse a good binder to a poor binder or enhance a poor binder to become a better binder. IC$_{50}$ of <100 nM indicates a good binder, whereas <50 nM indicates an excellent binder. These data are from study of binding of virus-specific MHC-restricted peptides to the appropriate MHC class I-D^b glycoprotein. See Hudrisier et al. 2001 for details.

(Fujinami and Oldstone 1985) (Fig. 2). Several myelin basic protein sequences that cause EAE are known, and the encephalitogenic site of 8 to 10 amino acids has been mapped for multiple animal species. The first step was computer analysis to match the myelin proteins (peptides) known to cause EAE to viral proteins for homologies. That search uncovered several such viral proteins, including a hemagglutinin nucleoprotein of influenza virus, the core protein

Table 2 Interesting sequence similarities between microbial proteins and human host proteins

Protein	Residue	Sequence
Measles virus P3	219	EISDNLGQEGRASTSGTP
Myelin basic protein	158	EISFKLGQEGRDSRSGTP
Measles virus P3	13	LECIRALK
Corticotropin	18	LECIRACK
Adenovirus 12 E1B	384	LRRGMFRPSQCN
A-gliadin	206	LGQGSFRPSQQN
Klebsiella pneumoniae nitrogenase	186	SRQTDREDE
Human lymphocyte antigen B27	70	KAZTDREDL
Rabies virus glycoprotein	147	TKESLVIIS
Insulin receptor	764	NKESLVISE
Papillomavirus E2	76	SLHLESLKDS
Insulin receptor	66	VYGLESLKDL
Poliovirus VP2	70	STTKESRGTT
Acetylcholine receptor	176	TVIKESRGTK
Coxsackie B3	2152	YEAFIRKIRSV
Myosin	138	YEAFVKHIMSV
Dengue	269	IKKSKAL
Coagulation factor x1	68	IKKSKAL
HIV Pol	222	DSTKWRKVD
Brain protein	156	DSTKNRKTD
HCMV IE-2	79	PDPLGRPDED
HLA DR	50	VTELGRPDAE

of adenovirus, the EC-LF2 protein of Epstein-Barr virus, the hepatitis B virus polymerase (HBVP), and several other viral proteins. The best fit was between the myelin basic protein encephalitogenic site in the rabbit and HBVP. Subsequently, inoculation of the HBVP peptide peripherally into rabbits caused perivascular infiltration localized to the central nervous system, reminiscent of the disease induced by inoculating whole myelin basic protein or the peptide component of the encephalitogenic site of myelin basic protein (Fujinami and Oldstone 1985) (Fig. 2). Furthermore, a specific immune response, both cellular and humoral, to myelin basic protein occurred. However this model was artificial, because there was no epidemiological evidence associating hepatitis

Biological Consequences of Mimicry Between Rabbit Myelin Basic Protein (MBP) and Hepatitis B Virus Polymerase (HBVP)

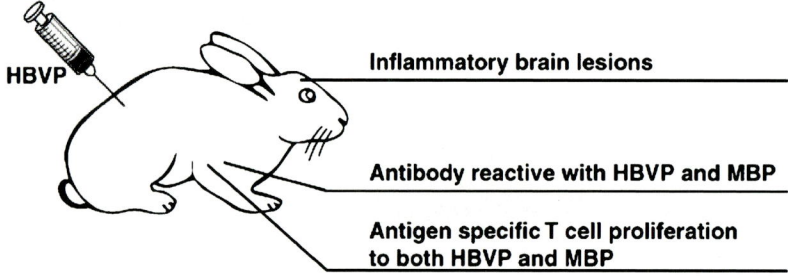

Fig. 2 First demonstration that molecular mimicry could cause disease. When New Zealand rabbits were inoculated with the 10-amino acid peptide from hepatitis B virus polymerase (*HBVP*), they generated specific T (proliferation) and B (antibody) lymphocyte responses. Most significant, inoculated rabbits developed histopathologic criteria for lesions of EAE. In contrast, studies with over 10 different peptides in multiple rabbits failed to elicit EAE. (See Fujinami and Oldstone 1985 for experimental details)

B with an EAE-like disease. Nevertheless, the importance of the observation was in providing proof of the molecular mimicry concept in vivo. A more meaningful model followed with our observations correlating several bacteria with HLA B27-associated ankylosing spondylitis (AS), an arthritic disease of humans. Epidemiological, bacteriologic, and immunologic evidence is firm for a strong relationship between AS, the hypervariable region of HLA B27, and several bacterial infections including those of *Shigella flexneri*, *Yersinia enterocolitica*, and *Klebsiella pneumoniae* (Brewerton et al. 1973; Gilliland and Mannik 1986; Khare et al. 1996; Schwimmbeck and Oldstone 1989). Over 90% of patients who develop AS have the HLA B27 haplotype, but this haplotype occurs in only about 10% of the general population. Further, monozygotic twins show a discordance for AS (Eastmond and Woodrow 1977), indicating a role for environmental factors, which epidemiological evidence suggests is associated with infections by selective bacteria. For example, in a *S. flexneri* epidemic of about 150,000 cases in Finland during the 1940s, 344 infected individuals developed Reiter's syndrome; of these 82 went on to develop AS. We observed amino acid sequence homology between enteric bacteria known to cause Reiter's syndrome and thus associated with AS and with the hypervariable region of HLA B27 (Table 2, Fig. 3).

To mimic AS, we humanized mice through transgenic technology to express human HLA (LaFace et al. 1995). For HLA B27-restricted T cell function, it was necessary to create a triple transgenic mouse that not only expressed human HLA B27 but also human β_2-microglobulin and human CD8 (Tishon et al. 2000). Challenge of such humanized transgenic mice with cross-reactive peptides derived from the bacteria (Fig. 3) led to immune responses with inflammatory cells located in the joints and vertebral columns of approximately

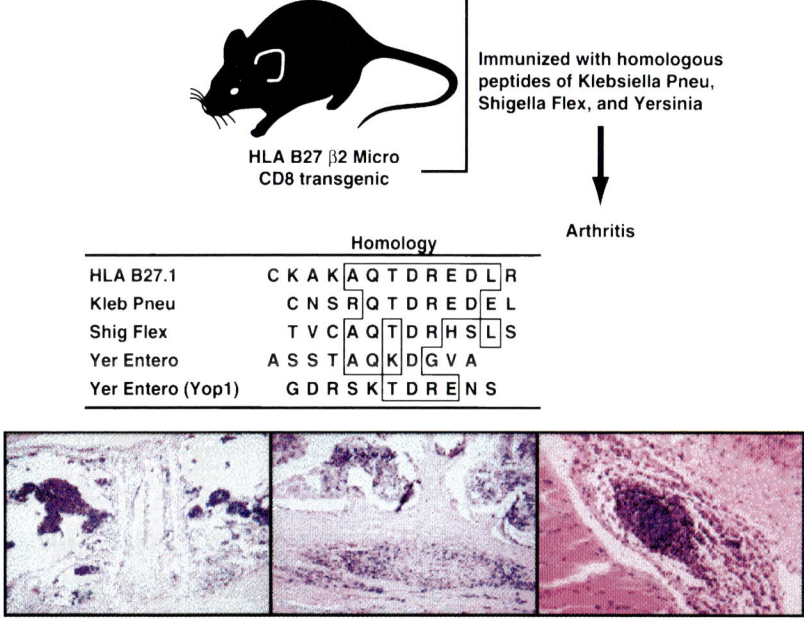

Fig. 3 Sequence sharing between the hypervariable region of HLA B27 molecule and sequences from bacteria epidemiologically associated with causing Reiter's syndrome, a disease that often precedes HLA B27-associated ankylosing spondylitis. Inoculation of the *Shigella flexneri* peptide (*center panel*) or *Klebsiella pneumoniae* peptide (*right panel*) into transgenic mice expressing HLA B27 human β2-microglobulin and human CD8 leads to inflammatory responses in joints and the vertebral column. Monoclonal antibodies to HLA B27 are also found in these mice, but not in other mice given cross-reactive bacterial peptides. The control mice also fail to demonstrate inflammatory lesions (*left panel*)

40% of the inoculated, triple transgenic mice but not of control mice (Oldstone 1998). Interestingly, a transgenic rat model was developed by Hammer et al. (1990) in which HLA B27 expression was associated with a clinical and histopathologic picture reminiscent of AS. AS-like disease occurred in rats housed in a normal vivarium but not when such rats were quartered under germ-free conditions (Taurog et al. 1994). Yet, when the germ-free rats were later colonized by bacteria, they developed arthritis (Rath et al. 1996). In addition to the molecular mimicry mechanism, HLA B27 may be associated with a delayed or disordered clearance of these bacterial pathogens.

Several other informative animal models were developed to show cross-reactivity between a microbe and self-antigen leading to autoimmune disease (reviewed in Cunningham and Fujinami 2000, Oldstone 1989, 1998). One interesting example is presented in publications from the laboratories of Harvey Cantor and Priscilla Schaffer (Zhao et al. 1997) for herpes simplex virus with corneal antigens. Others are reviewed in this volume. Steve Miller and his associates describe a Theiler's virus-induced molecular mimicry model of multiple sclerosis, whereas Larry Steinman and colleagues report on molecular mimicry and peptide protection of EAE. The last chapter in the series on animal models of infection is from my laboratory and focuses on the principles of how molecular mimicry works and the quantitation of cross-reactive antigen-specific T cells required for disease in a transgenic model of type I diabetes.

5
Equating Human Autoimmune Disease with Molecular Mimicry

The most difficult step in the process described here is to definitively prove the relevance of molecular mimicry to human autoimmune disease. Various correlations ranging from those that are reasonably convincing to those that are less so have been published (reviewed in Oldstone 1998). Two examples are selected for brief mention. The first is the autoimmune disease myasthenia gravis. The majority of these patients have antibodies against the acetylcholine receptor (AChR). Purification of antibodies from patients with myasthenia gravis using the human AChR α-subunit from amino acids 157 to 170 as a probe uncovered, as expected, immunoglobulin G antibodies that bound to native AChR and inhibited the binding of α-bungarotoxin to its receptor. In addition, the human AChR α-subunit from amino acids 160 to 167 showed specific immunologic cross-reactivity with a shared homologous domain on herpes simplex virus glycoprotein D, residues 286 to 293, by both specific binding and inhibition assays. Antibodies, including monoclonals, to the human AChR α-subunit bound to herpes simplex virus-infected cells (Schwimmbeck et al. 1989). The data on the immunologic cross-reactivity of the AChR "self-epitope" with herpes simplex virus and the presence of cross-reactive antibodies in the sera of patients with myasthenia gravis suggest the possibility that this virus may be associated with some cases of myasthenia gravis.

In another study, Wucherpfennig and Strominger (1995) imposed a structural requirement for molecular mimicry searches. These investigators used the known structures for MHC class II disease-associated molecules that bind to specific peptides and the T cell receptor for a known immunodominant myelin basic protein peptide. A database search produced a panel of 129 peptides from microbes that matched the molecular mimicry motif, and these were tested with several T cell clones obtained from the cerebrospinal fluid of patients with multiple sclerosis. Eight peptides (seven of viral origin and one of bacterial origin) were found to efficiently activate three of these clones. In contrast, only one of the eight peptides would have been identified as an appropriate molecular mimic by sequence alignment. These observations indicated that a single T cell receptor could recognize several distinct but structurally related peptides from multiple pathogens, suggesting more permissivity for the T cell receptor than has been previously appreciated (also see Mason 1998). This issue is further explored in this volume by K.W. Wucherpfennig.

In this volume, for additional studies of human disease, K. Bachmaier and J. Penninger review their body of work associating chlamydia-induced molecular mimicry and other microbial infections with immune responses to cardiac antigens and resultant heart disease; and John Stuart discusses HTLV-1-induced molecular mimicry and tropical sprue myelopathy. Betty Diamond presents recent provocative findings of molecular mimicry between anti-DNA antibodies and the NR2 glutamate receptor in systemic lupus erythematosus.

6
Overview of Autoimmune Responses and Infections

The autoimmune response is often a pathway of immunity that attacks one's own tissues and causes disease. Most autoimmune diseases are organ (tissue) specific, and they develop when lymphocytes or their products (cytokines, antibodies, perforin, etc.) react with a limited number of antigens in that tissue. The molecular mechanisms leading to autoreactive immune responses resemble those generated against foreign antigens such as bacteria, parasites, or viruses. However, in autoimmune disease either incomplete clonal deletion or formation of clonal anergy of T cells establishes a population of cells that is potentially intolerant but under special circumstances able to react with the host's antigens. Autoimmune disorders are, then, characterized by the breaking of immunologic tolerance or of unresponsiveness to self-antigens. What is the evidence suggesting that some infectious agents, primarily viruses, can similarly break immunologic tolerance and are thus implicated in autoimmune diseases?

The evidence suggesting the involvement of viruses or other infectious agents in human autoimmune diseases came initially from studies of identical twins that clearly implicated environmental factors as a cause, because genetic factors alone could not be responsible. Genetic studies in such autoimmune diseases as multiple sclerosis, diabetes, AS, etc., were complemented by epidemiological evidence incriminating local events (geography) or multiple infections with these diseases (Eastmond and Woodrow 1977; Ebers et al. 1987; Gamble 1980; Green 1990; Jury et al. 1996; Kurtzke 1993; Merriman and Todd 1995; Panitch 1994; Theofilopoulos 1995). Indeed, it is well known that newly forming autoimmune responses or those previously present are enhanced after infection by numerous human DNA and RNA viruses (reviewed in Oldstone 1998). In fact, after infection, patients can mount immune responses to nucleic acids, cytoskeletal proteins, myosin, and lymphocytes, etc., as shown over 45 years ago by the great Swedish immunologist Asterid Fagraeus. Additionally, experimental acute and persistent infections with a DNA or RNA virus have induced, accelerated, or enhanced autoimmune responses and caused autoimmune disease. The New Zealand mouse family is a genetically defined group in which certain strains spontaneously develop autoimmune disease. For example, among their several typical autoimmune responses, NZB mice develop antibodies to DNA and red blood cells, whereas NZB×NZW (F1) mice develop antibodies to DNA and other nuclear antigens, closely resembling the picture of humans with systemic lupus erythematosus. When NZB or (NZB×W) F1 mice are persistently infected with either a DNA (polyoma) or an RNA (lymphocytic choriomeningitis virus, LCMV) virus, their autoimmune responses occur earlier, reach higher titers, and lead to disease sooner than in their uninfected counterparts (Tonietti et al. 1970). More interestingly, NZW mice compared to NZB and (NZB×W) F1 mice normally have no or only moderate autoimmune responses. However, NZW mice contain the necessary gene(s) for autoimmune disease and develop markedly accelerated autoimmune responses and acquire a lupus-like disease after infection by polyoma virus or LCMV. Other viruses, including retroviruses, cause a similar phenomenon. In human autoimmune diseases like multiple sclerosis, insulin-dependent diabetes mellitus (IDDM), or AS, the incidence of disease varies in monozygotic twins, again indicating that other factors, in addition to genetics and most likely environmental, play a role (Green 1990; Jury et al. 1996; Merriman and Todd 1995; Oldstone 1998; Theofilopoulos 1995). Some have observed that infectious agents or cytokines released in the presence and/or absence of preexisting infections can break tolerance in potentially autoreactive $CD4^+$ T or $CD8^+$ T cells. Others have reported epidemiological and serological correlations between certain viruses and autoimmune diseases like multiple sclerosis (Ebers et al. 1987; Kurtzke 1993; Panitch 1994) and IDDM (Gamble 1980; Honeyman et al. 1998; Notkins and Yoon 1984). For example, Coxsackie B virus and rubella virus have been linked with IDDM. In a few instances, Coxsackie B virus has been directly isolated from pancreatic tissues of individuals with acute IDDM. Inoculation of this virus into mice then produced IDDM, fulfilling Koch's postulates (Yoon et al. 1989), although this occurrence is rare.

7
Summary

In conclusion, molecular mimicry is but one mechanism by which autoimmune diseases can occur in association with infectious agents. The concept of molecular mimicry remains a viable hypothesis for framing questions and approaches to uncovering the initiating infectious agent as well as recognizing the "self"-determinant, understanding the pathogenic mechanism(s) involved, and designing strategies for the treatment and prevention of autoimmune disorders. The *Oxford Dictionary* defines hypothesis as "a supposition or conjecture put forward to account for certain facts and used as a basis for further investigation by which it may be proved or disproved." In many instances, hard data derived in experimental systems clearly indicate molecular mimicry as a mechanism for disease causation. For others, especially human disorders, the evidence can be strongly suggestive, but additional information is required before molecular mimicry can be accepted or rejected as biological reality. The availability of computer data banks, structural information on specific MHC alleles, and MHC maps for particular autoimmune diseases is crucial for answering such questions. Further, the ability to identify anchoring and flanking sequences of a peptide that binds to the MHC allele or T cell receptor in question provides the opportunity to better identify the microbial causes of autoimmune diseases. The application and use of transgenic models designed to evaluate molecular mimicry enable us to understand the sequence of events that leads to the related pathological effects as well as to design specific and unique therapies that can reverse or prevent the autoimmune destructive process.

Acknowledgements This is Publication Number 16970-NP from the Departments of Neuropharmacology and Infectology, The Scripps Research Institute, La Jolla, CA. This work was supported in the past and currently in part by USPHS Grants DK-058541, AI-009484, AI-045927, and AI-036222.

References

Atkinson MA, Bowman MA, Campbell L, Darrow BL, Kaufman DL, MacLaren NK (1994) Cellular immunity to a determinant common to glutamate decarboxylase and coxsackie virus in insulin-dependent diabetes. J Clin Invest 94:2125–2129

Bachmaier K, Neu N, de la Maza LM, Pal S, Hessel A, Penninger JM (1999) Chlamydia infections and heart disease linked through antigenic mimicry. Science 283:1335–1339

Brewerton D, Caffrey M, Hart F, James D, Nichols A, Sturrock R (1973) Ankylosing spondylitis and HLA B27. Lancet i:904–907

Cunningham MW (2004) T cell mimicry in inflammatory heart disease. Mol Immunol 40:1121–1127

Cunningham MW, Fujinami RS (eds) (2000) Molecular mimicry. ASM Press, Washington DC

Dales S, Fujinami RS, Oldstone MBA (1983a) Serologic relatedness between Thy1.2 and actin revealed by monoclonal antibody. J Immunol 131:1332–1338

Dales S, Fujinami RS, Oldstone MBA (1983b) Infection with vaccinia favors the selection of hybridomas synthesizing auto-antibodies against intermediate filaments, among them one cross-reacting with the virus hemagglutinin. J Immunol 131:1546–1553

Dell A, Antone SM, Gauntt CJ, Crossley CA, Clark WA, Cunningham MW (1991) Autoimmune determinants of rheumatic carditis: localization of epitopes in human cardiac myosin. Eur Heart J 12:158–162

Dixon FJ (1963) The role of antigen antibody complexes in disease. Harvey Lecture 58:21–52

Dyrberg T, Oldstone MBA (1986) Peptides as probes to study molecular mimicry and virus-induced autoimmunity. Curr Topics Microbiol Immunol 130:25–37

Dyrberg T, Petersen JS, Oldstone MBA (1990) Immunological cross-reactivity between mimicking epitopes on a virus protein and a human autoantigen depends on a single amino acid residue. Clin Immunol Immunopathol 54:290–297

Eastmond CJ, Woodrow JC (1977) Discordance for ankylosing spondylitis in monozygotic twins. Ann Rheum Dis 36:360

Ebers G, Bulman D, Sadovnik A, Paty DW, Warren S, Hader W, Murray TJ, Seland TP, Duquette P, Grey T et al. (1987) A population-based study of multiple sclerosis in twins. N Engl J Med 315:1638–1642

Froude J, Gibofsky A, Buskirk DR, Khana A, Zabriskie JB (1989) Reactivity between streptococcus and human tissue. Curr Topics Microbiol Immunol 145:5–26

Fujinami RS, Oldstone MBA (1985) Amino acid homology between the encephalitogenic site of myelin basic protein and virus: Mechanism for autoimmunity. Science 230:1043–1045

Fujinami RS, Oldstone MBA, Wroblewska Z, Frankel ME, Koprowski H (1983) Molecular mimicry in virus infection: cross-reaction of measles phosphoprotein or of herpes simplex virus protein with human intermediate filaments. Proc Natl Acad Sci USA 80:2346–2350

Gamble DR (1980) The epidemiology of insulin-dependent diabetes with particular reference to the relationship of virus infection to its etiology. Epidemiol Rev 2:49–70

Gilliland B, Mannik M (1986) Ankylosing spondylitis and Reiter's syndrome (pp 1986–1988) and rheumatoid arthritis (pp 1977–1986). In: Harrison TR (ed) Harrison's Principles of Internal Medicine, 10th Edition. McGraw Hill, New York

Green A (1990) The role of genetic factors in development of IDDM. Curr Topics Microbiol Immunol 164:3–17

Hafer-Macko C, Hsieh ST, Li CY, Ho TW, Sheikh K, Cornblath DR, McKhann GM, Asbury AK, Griffin JW (1996) Acute motor axonal neuropathy: an antibody-mediated attack on axolemma. Ann Neurol 40:635–644

Hammer RE, Maika SD, Richardson JA, Tang JP, Taurog JD (1990) Spontaneous inflammatory disease in transgenic mice expressing HLA-B27 and human β2m: an animal model of HLA-B27-associated human disorders. Cell 63:1099–1112

Honeyman MC, Stone NL, Harrison LC (1998) T-cell epitopes in type 1 diabetes autoantigen tyrosine phosphatase IA-2: potential for mimicry with rotavirus and other environmental agents. Mol Med 4:231–239

Hudrisier D, Riond J, Burlet-Schiltz O, von Herrath MB, Lewicki H, Monsarrat B, Oldstone MBA, Gairin JE (2001) Structural and functional identification of major histocompatibility complex class I-restricted self-peptides as naturally occurring molecular mimics of viral antigens. J Biol Chem 276:19396–19403

Jury KM, Loeffler D, Eiermann TH, Ziegler B, Boehm BO, Richter W (1996) Evidence for somatic mutation and affinity maturation of diabetes associated human autoantibodies to glutamate decarboxylase. J Autoimmun 9:371–377

Kaplan MH (1963) Immunologic reactivity of streptococcal and tissue antigens. J Immunol 90:595–606

Khare SD, Luthra HS, David CS (1996) Role of HLA-B27 in spondyloarthropathies. Curr Topics Microbiol Immunol 206:85–97

Kurtzke JF (1993) Epidemiologic evidence for multiple sclerosis as an infection. Clin Microbiol Rev 6:382–427

LaFace DM, Vestberg M, Yang Y, Srivastava R, DiSanto J, Flomenberg N, Brown S, Sherman LA, Peterson PA (1995) Human CD8 transgene regulation of HLA recognition by murine T cells. J Exp Med 182:1315–1325

Lane DP, Hoeffler WK (1980) SV40 large T shares an antigenic determinant with a cellular protein of molecular weight 68,000. Nature 288:167–170

Mason D (1998) A very high level of crossreactivity is an essential feature of the T-cell receptor. Immunol Today 19:395–404

Merriman TR, Todd JA (1995) Genetics of autoimmune disease. Curr Opin Immunol 7:786–792

Notkins AL, Yoon JW (1984) Virus-induced diabetes mellitus. In: Notkins AL, Oldstone MBA (eds) Concepts in Viral Pathogenesis. Springer-Verlag, New York, pp 241–247

Oldstone MBA (1987) Molecular mimicry and autoimmune disease. Cell 50:819–820

Oldstone MBA (ed) (1989) Molecular mimicry. Curr Topics Microbiol Immunol, Vol. 145
Oldstone MBA (1998) Molecular mimicry and immune-mediated diseases. FASEB J 12:1255–1265
Oldstone MBA, von Herrath M, Lewicki H, Hudrisier D, Whitton JL, Gairin JE (1999) Use of a high-affinity peptide that aborts MHC-restricted cytotoxic T lymphocyte activity against multiple viruses in vitro and virus-induced immunopathologic disease in vivo. Virology 256:246–257
Panitch HS (1994) Influence of infection on exacerbations of multiple sclerosis. Ann Neurol 36:S25
Rath HC, Herfarth HH, Ikeda JS, Grenther WB, Hamm TE Jr, Balish E, Taurog JD, Hammer RE, Wilson KH, Sartor RB (1996) Normal luminal bacteria, especially Bacteroides species, mediate chronic colitis, gastritis, and arthritis in HLA-B27/human beta2 microglobulin transgenic rates. J Clin Invest 98:945–953
Schwimmbeck P, Oldstone MBA (1989) *Klebsiella pneumoniae* and HLA B27 associated diseases of Reiter's syndrome and ankylosing spondylitis. Curr Topics Microbiol Immunol 145:45–67
Schwimmbeck PL, Dyrberg T, Drachman D, Oldstone MBA (1989) Molecular mimicry and myasthenia gravis: An autoantigenic site of the acetylcholine receptor α-subunit that has biologic activity and reacts immunochemically with herpes simplex virus. J Clin Invest 84:1174–1180
Schwimmbeck PL, Yu DTY, Oldstone MBA (1987) Autoantibodies to HLA B27 in the sera of HLA B27 patients with ankylosing spondylitis and Reiter's syndrome: Molecular mimicry with Klebsiella pneumoniae as potential mechanism of autoimmune disease. J Exp Med 166:173–181
Shrinivasappa J, Saegusa J, Prabhakar B, Gentry M, Buchmeier M, Wiktor T, Koprowski H, Oldstone M, Notkins A (1986) Molecular mimicry: frequency of reactivity of monoclonal antiviral antibodies with normal tissues. J Virol 57:397–401
Taurog JD, Richardson JA, Croft JT, Simmons WA, Zhou M, Fernandez-Sueiro JL, Balish E, Hammer RE (1994) The germfree state prevents development of gut and joint inflammatory disease in HLA-B27 transgenic mice. J Exp Med 180:2359–2364
Theofilopoulos A (1995) The basis of autoimmunity. II. Genetic predisposition. Immunol Today 16:150–159
Tishon A, LaFace DM, Lewicki H, van Binnendijk RS, Osterhaus A, Oldstone MBA (2000) Transgenic mice expressing human HLA and CD8 molecules generate HLA-restricted measles virus cytotoxic T lymphocytes of the same specificity as humans with natural measles virus infection. Virology 275:286–293
Tonietti G, Oldstone MBA, Dixon FJ (1970) The effect of induced chronic viral infections on the immunologic diseases of New Zealand mice. J Exp Med 132:89–109
Wucherpfennig KW, Strominger JL (1995) Molecular mimicry in T-cell mediated autoimmunity: viral peptides activate human T-cell clones specific for myelin basic protein. Cell 80:695–705
Yoon JW, Austin M, Onodera T, Notkins AL (1989) Virus-induced diabetes mellitus: isolation of a virus from the pancreas of a child with diabetic ketoacidosis. N Engl J Med 300:1173–1179

Yuki N, Susuki K, Koga M, Nishimoto Y, Odaka M, Hirata K, Taguchi K, Miyatake T, Furukawa K, Kobata T, Yamada M (2004) Carbohydrate mimicry between human ganglioside GM1 and *Campylobacter jejuni* lipooligosaccharide causes Guillain-Barre syndrome. Proc Natl Acad Sci USA 101:11404–11409

Zhao ZS, Granucci F, Yeh L, Schaffer P, Cantor H (1997) Molecular mimicry by herpes simplex virus type 1: autoimmune disease after viral infection. Science 79:1344–1347

The Structural Interactions Between T Cell Receptors and MHC–Peptide Complexes Place Physical Limits on Self–Nonself Discrimination

K. W. Wucherpfennig (✉)

Department of Cancer Immunology and AIDS, Dana-Farber Cancer Institute, 44 Binney Street, Boston, MA 02115, USA
wucherpf@mbcrr.harvard.edu

1	How Specific Is TCR Recognition of MHC–Peptide Complexes?	20
2	Development of a Strategy to Systematically Examine TCR Cross-Reactivity	22
3	T Cell Clones Can Recognize Multiple Peptides with Limited Sequence Similarity	22
4	Activation of MBP-Specific T Cells by Naturally Processed Viral Antigen	23
5	Crystal Structure of the HLA-DR2–MBP Peptide Complex	24
6	Common Features of Microbial Peptides That Activate MBP-Specific T Cells	26
7	Structural Features of Autoreactive TCRs That Contribute to the Degree of Cross-Reactivity	29
8	TCR Cross-Reactivity and Immunopathology	31
9	TCR Cross-Reactivity as a General Property of T Cell Recognition	32
References		34

Abstract The activation and expansion of T cells in an antimicrobial immune response is based on the ability of T cell receptors (TCR) to discriminate between MHC-bound peptides derived from different microbial agents as well as self-proteins. However, the specificity of T cells is constrained by the limited number of peptide side chains that are available for TCR binding. By considering the structural requirements for peptide binding to MHC molecules and TCR recognition of MHC–peptide complexes, we demonstrated that human T cell clones could recognize a number of peptides from different organisms that were remarkably distinct in their primary sequence. These peptides were particularly diverse at those sequence positions buried in pockets of the MHC binding site, whereas a higher degree of similarity was present at a limited number of peptide residues that created the interface with the TCR. These T cell clones had been isolated from multiple sclerosis patients with human myelin basic protein, demonstrating that activation of such autoreactive T cells by microbial peptides with sufficient structural similarity may contribute to the disease process. Similar findings have now been made for a variety of human and murine T cell clones, indicating that specificity and cross-reactivity are inherent properties of TCR recognition. The observations that particular TCR are highly sensitive to changes at particular peptide positions but insensitive to many other changes in peptide sequence are not contradictory, but rather the result of structural interactions in which a relatively flat TCR surface contacts a limited number of side chains from a peptide that is deeply embedded in the MHC binding site.

1
How Specific Is TCR Recognition of MHC–Peptide Complexes?

The experimental practice of isolating "antigen-specific" T cells by in vivo or in vitro selection with a particular antigen led to the widely held notion that T cell receptor (TCR) recognition is highly specific because T cell clones selected in such a fashion are typically not activated by control antigens. Within this conceptual framework it was thought that rare microbial antigens in which the peptide sequences were closely related to a self-peptide could represent mimics responsible for the induction of autoimmune diseases. Sequence alignment between an encephalitogenic epitope of myelin basic protein (MBP) and microbial proteins permitted identification of a peptide from the hepatitis B virus DNA polymerase that induced histological signs of experimental autoimmune encephalomyelitis (EAE) after immunization of rabbits (Fujinami and Oldstone 1985). Subsequently, many investigators used sequence alignments to identify potential mimicry peptides, but the vast majority of peptides had no biological activity. It thus appeared that TCR cross-reactivity might be a very rare event. Given the paucity of definitive experimental data, the biological relevance of TCR cross-reactivity was questioned by many basic scientists.

However, structural studies on the interaction of MHC molecules with peptides and on TCR recognition of MHC–peptide complexes suggested that this view of TCR recognition might have to be reconsidered. Peptide elution studies demonstrated that a single MHC molecule could bind a very large and diverse set of peptides because several hundred distinct peptide masses could be defined with mass spectrometry techniques (Hunt et al. 1992; Chicz et al. 1993). Investigation of the structural requirements for peptide binding by MHC class II molecules demonstrated that five peptide side chains contributed to binding (Stern et al. 1994). However, each of these "anchor residues" could typically be substituted by a number of other amino acids so that the resulting peptide binding motifs were highly degenerate (Hammer et al. 1993). For the multiple sclerosis (MS)-associated HLA-DR2 molecule (DRA, DRB1*1501) that has been the focus of our studies, three of these five peptide positions (P6, P7, and P9 pockets) could be substituted by many different amino acids. Even though a higher degree of specificity was observed for the P1 and P4 anchor residues, substitutions by structurally related amino acids were permitted (Wucherpfennig et al. 1994a). The crystal structure of HLA-DR1 with a bound peptide from influenza hemagglutinin (HA, 306–318) elucidated how peptides are bound with high affinity, despite such degenerate sequence motifs: A significant fraction of the binding energy is derived from interactions between the backbone of the peptide and conserved residues of the MHC class II binding cleft. This structure also demonstrated that the peptide is buried in the binding site such that substitutions of peptide side chains located in deep pockets might not interfere with TCR recognition of the MHC–peptide surface (Stern et al. 1994).

Analysis of TCR recognition of MHC-bound peptides in light of this structural information demonstrated that specificity was typically confined to a small number of peptide side chains. For the MBP-specific T cell clones that we have studied, three peptide side chains in the core of the MBP peptide (P2 His, P3 Phe, and P5 Lys) were particularly relevant for TCR recognition (Wucherpfennig et al. 1994a; Wucherpfennig and Strominger 1995). This observation appeared to be general because similar findings were made for murine TCR reactive with microbial or self-antigens. Global amino acid replacements in the moth cytochrome C (93–103) peptide recognized by murine I-E^k restricted T cells demonstrated a strong preference for a particular amino acid at three peptide positions (Reay et al. 1994). For the Ac(1–11) peptide of MBP that is encephalitogenic in PL/J mice, only four native MBP residues were required for activation of MBP-specific T cells (Gautam et al. 1994).

On the basis of these considerations, we developed the hypothesis that TCR recognition is characterized by a considerable degree of cross-reactivity and that a TCR could recognize a number of different peptides that may be rather distinct in their sequence. This hypothesis was supported by a reported case of cross-reactivity where no obvious sequence similarity was present between the two peptides, as well as the observation that many T cell clones recognized alloreactive MHC–peptide complexes (Bhardwaj et al. 1993; Burrows et al. 1994).

2
Development of a Strategy to Systematically Examine TCR Cross-Reactivity

The challenge therefore was to develop a systematic approach that would allow us to identify such peptides even though their structural similarity might not be evident by conventional sequence alignments. Formation of the trimolecular complex of MHC, peptide, and TCR is based on two independent binding events: high-affinity binding of peptide to an MHC molecule and the more short-lived association of TCR with this MHC–peptide surface. We decided to base our strategy on the minimal structural requirements for each of these two binding events. This approach took advantage of the fact that T cell epitopes can be mapped to short peptide segments and that the contribution of individual peptide side chains to MHC binding and TCR recognition can be evaluated with a series of peptide analogs. Experimentally, this work focused on T cell recognition of a peptide from human MBP (residues 85–99) that is bound with high affinity by the multiple sclerosis (MS)-associated HLA-DR2 molecule (DRA, DRB1*1501) (Wucherpfennig et al. 1994a). Analysis of TCR cross-reactivity for T cell clones activated by this HLA-DR2/MBP peptide complex could thus provide insights into disease mechanisms in MS. We defined the minimal structural requirements for binding of the MBP peptide to HLA-DR2 and for TCR recognition of this MHC–peptide complex and searched available sequence databases with this motif information. This approach permitted the identification of many examples of TCR cross-reactivity, not only for the human MBP-specific T cell clones that we have studied but also for CD4 and CD8 T cells of both human and murine origin, as described in some of the other chapters in this volume. A more recent variant of this approach has been to determine the search motif with peptide analogs in which all neighboring positions carry mixtures of amino acids (so-called combinatorial peptide libraries/positional scanning libraries) (Hemmer et al. 1997). These libraries provide less detailed motif information but can be used on any MHC class II restricted T cell clone.

3
T Cell Clones Can Recognize Multiple Peptides with Limited Sequence Similarity

The search criteria focused on the two major HLA-DR2 anchor residues of the peptide (P1 and P4) and four putative TCR contact residues (at P -1, P2, P3, and P5), all of which were located in a six-amino acid core segment of the peptide. In the initial study, we synthesized a panel of 129 microbial peptides that matched these criteria and tested them for their ability to activate human MBP-specific T cell clones that had been isolated from the peripheral blood of two patients with MS. Even though we only analyzed T cell clones that recognized a single self-peptide, we could identify eight microbial peptides that activated MBP-reactive T cell clones (Wucherpfennig and Strominger 1995). These peptides were remarkably distinct in their sequence from each other and the MBP peptide, and only one of the eight peptides had obvious sequence similarity with the MBP peptide in the core segment. The motif-based strategy was thus essential for the identification of these peptides. In the initial study, such peptides were identified for three of the seven T cell clones that we studied. To determine whether microbial peptides could activate the majority of these clones, we examined the recognition motif for two of the four remaining clones in detail and synthesized a panel of peptides that included sequences from recently characterized microbial genomes. A total of five bacterial peptides were identified in this set of experiments (Hausmann et al. 1999a). Thus we have identified a total of 13 microbial peptides that can activate human T cell clones specific for a single myelin peptide. Because we could only synthesize a subset of peptides identified in each search and a number of microbial genomes have not yet been sequenced, it is evident that a substantial number of microbial peptides can activate T cell clones that recognize this MBP peptide. These experiments thus demonstrated that T cell clones could recognize a variety of different peptides with limited sequence similarity.

A number of different terms have been used to describe this property of TCR recognition. TCR cross-reactivity describes the basic biological observation, and plasticity and degeneracy suggest structural mechanisms—mobility of TCR CDR loops (plasticity) or a relatively poor fit of the TCR on the MHC–peptide surface (degeneracy). Molecular mimicry has been widely used to describe the specialized case in which TCR cross-reactivity involves peptides from an infectious agent and a self-antigen.

4
Activation of MBP-Specific T Cells by Naturally Processed Viral Antigen

One of the viral peptides was derived from the EBV DNA polymerase, and we examined whether the viral peptide is presented by infected antigen-presenting cells to MBP-specific T cells. The EBV DNA polymerase gene is part of the lytic cycle and is therefore not transcribed in EBV-transformed B cells. However, the lytic cycle and expression of the EBV DNA polymerase gene can be induced by treatment of EBV-transformed B cells with phorbol esters (Datta et al. 1980). A HLA-DR2$^+$ B cell line that had been treated with a phorbol ester activated a MBP-specific T cell clone that recognized both MBP and EBV DNA polymerase peptides. T cell activation was blocked by a mAb specific for HLA-DR, but not by a control mAb against HLA-DQ, and was not observed when MHC-mismatched EBV-transformed B cells were used as antigen-presenting cells. These results demonstrated that the MBP-specific T cell clone recognized not only the EBV peptide but also antigen-presenting cells in which the viral gene was transcribed (Wucherpfennig and Strominger 1995).

5
Crystal Structure of the HLA-DR2–MBP Peptide Complex

Because the peptides that can be recognized by the same TCR are quite distinct in their primary sequence, an important question relates to the structural basis of TCR cross-reactivity. Structural information is also required to determine why only a subset of peptides that match the MHC binding/TCR recognition motif activate the appropriate T cell clones. We determined the crystal structure of HLA-DR2 (DRA, DRB1*1501) with the bound MBP peptide as a step toward defining molecular mimicry at a structural level (Smith et al. 1998). Figure 1 gives an overview of the structure and illustrates features of HLA-DR2 that are important for MBP peptide binding as well as TCR recognition of the HLA-DR2-MBP peptide complex. The MBP peptide is bound in an extended conformation as a type II polyproline helix, and MBP peptide side chains occupy the P1, P4, P6, and P9 pockets of the binding groove (Fig. 1A). The two major anchor residues of the MBP peptide (Val and Phe) occupy the P1 and P4 pockets of HLA-DR2. The P4 pocket of HLA-DR2 is distinct from DR molecules associated with other autoimmune diseases. In HLA-DR2, this pocket is large and predominantly hydrophobic because of the presence of a small residue (Ala) at a key polymorphic position (DRβ 71), which permits an aromatic side chain of the MBP peptide to be accommodated (Phe) (Fig. 1C). The peptide residues shown to be important for TCR recognition of the MBP peptide (P2 His, P3 Phe, and P5 Lys) are solvent exposed in the structure of the HLA-DR2-MBP peptide complex (Fig. 1B, D; Fig. 2). The recently determined structure of the complex of a human MBP-specific TCR (Ob.1A 12 TCR) and HLA-DR2/MBP demonstrated an unusual topology in which the TCR was shifted to the peptide N-terminus. Rather than being centered over the P5 peptide residue as in the structures involving microbial peptides (Garboczi et al., 1996; Ding et al., 1998; Hennecke et al., 2000), the CDR3 loops

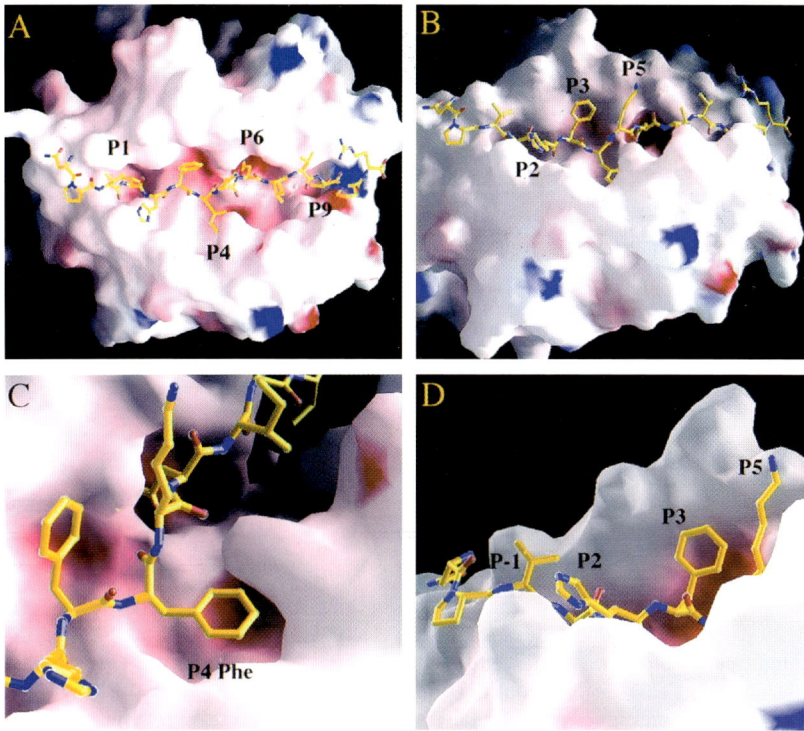

Fig. 1A–D Crystal structure of the complex of HLA-DR2 (DRA, DRB1*1501) and the MBP (85–99) peptide. **A** Overview of the structure. MBP peptide side chains that are located in four pockets of the binding site are indicated: P1 Val, P4 Phe, P6 Asn, and P9 Thr. **B** Solvent-exposed residues that are important for TCR recognition of the MBP (85–99) peptide: P2 His, P3 Phe, and P5 Lys. **C** P4 pocket of the HLA-DR2 binding site. This large and hydrophobic pocket is occupied by P4 Phe of the MBP peptide. The necessary room for this aromatic side chain is created by the presence of a small residue (Ala) at the polymorphic DRβ 71 position. **D** Close-up view of MBP peptide residues recognized by the TCR of MBP reactive T cell clones: P-1 Val, P2 His, P3 Phe, and P5 Lys. Preferences at these positions were considered in the search criteria for the identification of microbial peptides that activate MBP-reactive T cell clones. (Reprinted from *The Journal of Experimental Medicine*, Smith et al. 1998, with permission of the publisher)

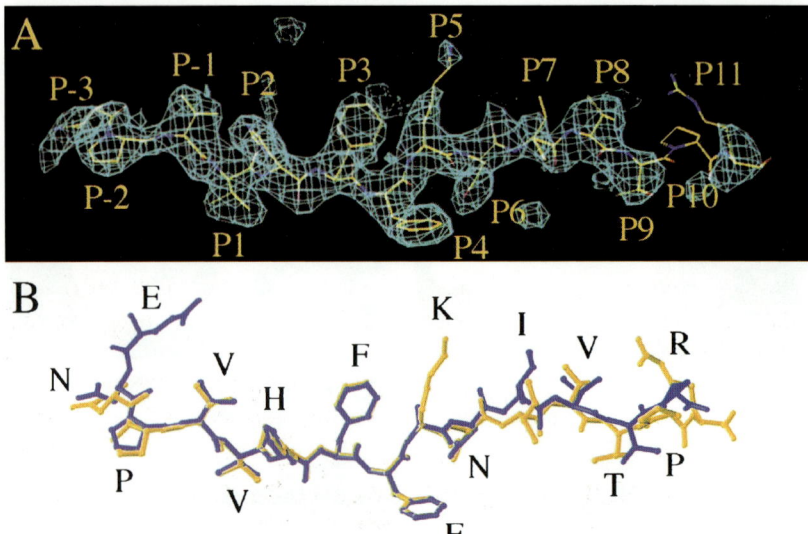

Fig. 2A, B Electron density and model of the MBP peptide in the binding site of HLA-DR2. A Experimental electron density of the MBP peptide bound to HLA-DR2. B. Model of the MBP peptide based on the electron density. The DR2-MBP peptide complex crystallized as a dimer of dimers, as other HLA-DR molecules (Brown et al. 1993; Stern et al. 1994), and both peptide copies are shown (*blue* and *yellow*). The peptide backbones superimpose in the P1 to P4 segment and are more divergent in the C-terminal segment because of different crystal contacts. (Reprinted from *The Journal of Experimental Medicine*, Smith et al. 1998, with permission of the publisher)

of TCRα and TCRβ are centered over P2 His of the MBP peptide (Hahn et al., 2005; see book cover). These results provide a potential mechanism for the escape of these T cells from thymic negative selection.

6
Common Features of Microbial Peptides That Activate MBP-Specific T Cells

The structural information on the HLA-DR2–MBP peptide complex was used to dissect the cross-reactive peptides identified for the MBP-specific T cell clone (Ob.1A12) for which the largest number of stimulatory microbial peptides were identified. The cross-reactive peptides were aligned with the MBP peptide in order to determine residues that may be located in pockets of the HLA-DR2 binding site (Table 1). This analysis shows that the HLA-DR2 con-

Table 1 Sequences of microbial peptides that activate human MBP-specific T cell clones

Peptides that activate T cell clone Ob.1A12 (HLA-DR2 restricted)

Organism	Source protein	Sequence
Homo sapiens	Myelin basic protein	ENPV**VHF**FKNIVTPR
Staphylococcus aureus	VgaB	VLARL**HF**YR**N**DVHKE
Mycobacterium avium	Transposase	QRCR**VHF**LR**N**VLAQV
Mycobacterium tuberculosis	Transposase	QRCR**VHF**MR**N**LYTAV
Bacillus subtilis	YqeE	ALA**VLHF**YPDKGAKN
Haemophilus influenzae/ *Escherichia coli*	HI0136/ORF	DFAR**VHF**ISALHGSG

Peptides that activate T cell clone Hy.1B11 (HLA-DQ1 restricted)

Organism	Source protein	Sequence
Homo sapiens	Myelin basic protein	ENPV**VHF**FKNIVTPR
Herpes simplex virus type 1	UL15 protein	FRQL**VHF**VRDFAQLL
Adenovirus type 12	ORF	DFE**VVT**FLKDVLPEF
Human papillomavirus type 7	L2 protein	IGGR**VHFFKD**ISPIA
Pseudomonas aeruginosa	Phosphomannomutase	DRLLML**FAKD**VVSRN

Microbial peptides that activate two human T cell clones reactive with the MBP (85–99) peptide are shown. Clone Ob.1A12 is restricted by HLA-DR2 (DRA, DRB1*1501), and five microbial peptides have been identified that activate this T cell clone. Clone Hy.1B11 is HLA-DQ1 restricted and activated by four microbial peptides that are quite distinct in their primary sequence. The peptide from human papillomavirus type 7 is the only peptide with obvious sequence similarity to the MBP peptide within the entire set of identified microbial peptides. Residues that are identical between the MBP peptide and microbial peptides are in bold. The HLA-DQ1-restricted T cell clone recognizes the same core segment of the MBP peptide as HLA-DR2-restricted clones (Wucherpfennig and Strominger 1995; Wucherpfennig et al. 1994a; Hausmann et al. 1999a). ORF, open reading frame.

tact surface of this set of peptides is highly diverse. No sequence identity with the MBP peptide is required on the HLA-DR2 binding surface, as illustrated by comparison of the MBP and *Bacillus subtilis* peptides. Common features of putative HLA-DR2 contact residues are the presence of an aliphatic residue in the P1 pocket and a large hydrophobic residue in the P4 pocket. At P6, a preference for asparagine is observed, whereas the residues that occupy the P7 and P9 positions are diverse. These data are in agreement with HLA-DR2 binding studies, which indicated that only two positions of the peptide (P1 and P4) were critical for binding and that they could be substituted with other aliphatic residues or phenylalanine (P1 pocket) or other hydrophobic residues (P4 pocket).

Analysis of the residues that may be solvent exposed and that could interact with the TCR shows a higher degree of sequence similarity/identity, in particular in the center of the epitope (Table 2). All peptides that activate this T cell clone carry the two primary TCR contact residues of the MBP peptide (His and Phe at P2 and P3). Also, a preference for a positively charged residue (Lys and Arg) is observed at P5. A high degree of sequence diversity is observed in the N- and C-terminal flanking segments, even though they are required

Table 2 Alignment of microbial peptides based on the crystal structure of the HLA-DR2–MBP peptide complex

Residues located in HLA-DR2 binding pockets

		1 4 67 9
Homo sapiens	Myelin basic protein	- - - -**V**- -**F**-**NI**-**T**- -
Staphylococcus aureus	VgaB	- - - -**L**- -Y-**ND**-H- -
Mycobacterium avium	Transposase	- - - -**V**- -L-**NV**-A- -
Mycobacterium tuberculosis	Transposase	- - - -**V**- -M-**NL**-**T**- -
Bacillus subtilis	YqeE	- - - -**L**- -Y-**DK**-A- -
Haemophilus influenzae/ *Escherichia coli*	HI0136/ORF	- - - -**V**- -I-**AL**-G- -

Solvent-exposed residues

		23 5 8
Homo sapiens	Myelin basic protein	**ENPV**-**HF**-**K**- -**V**-**PR**
Staphylococcus aureus	VgaB	VLAR-**HF**-R- -**V**-KE
Mycobacterium avium	Transposase	QRCR-**HF**-R- -L-QV
Mycobacterium tuberculosis	Transposase	QRCR-**HF**-R- -Y-AV
Bacillus subtilis	YqeE	ALAV-**HF**-P- -G-KN
Haemophilus influenzae/ *Escherichia coli*	HI0136/ORF	DFAR-**HF**-S- -H-SG

Peptide sequences were dissected in terms of putative HLA-DR2 anchor residues and solvent accessible residues that are available for interaction with the TCR. The HLA-DR2 contact surface of these peptides is highly diverse, and no sequence identity is observed at these five positions between the MBP and *Bacillus subtilis* peptides. A higher degree of sequence similarity/identity is observed for peptide residues that are likely to interact with the TCR (P2, P3, and P5). Numbers above the sequences represent positions in a nine-amino acid peptide core, starting with the anchor residue for the P1 pocket of the binding site.

for efficient T cell stimulation. The recent structure of the Ob.1A12 TCR bound to HLA-DR2/MBP explains these findings: only two TCR loops contact side chains of the HLA-DR2 bound MBP peptide (Hahn et al., 2005). This TCR therefore forms a smaller interfaction surface with the peptide than the influenza virus hemmagglutinin-specific HA 1.7 TCR (Hennecke et al., 2000).

The data also indicate that combinatorial effects shape the peptide surface that can be recognized by a TCR. Analysis of double-amino acid substitutions of the MBP peptide demonstrated that certain combinations of amino acids at TCR contact residues were stimulatory, even though the individual analogs had no activity (Ausubel et al. 1996). This notion is supported by the observation that the majority of microbial peptides that match the MHC binding/TCR recognition motif did not stimulate the MBP-specific T cell clones. Identification of a complete set of peptide sequences that represent agonists for a TCR will therefore require analysis of complex peptide libraries. At present, such analyses represent a technical challenge because a large number of peptides may need to be sequenced from phage display libraries or peptide libraries on beads. However, the complexity of the peptide repertoire that is recognized by an individual TCR may be underestimated unless the combinatorial nature of peptide recognition by the TCR is taken into consideration.

7
Structural Features of Autoreactive TCRs That Contribute to the Degree of Cross-Reactivity

Comparison of the MBP (85–99)-reactive T cell clones demonstrated obvious differences in the degree of specificity/cross-reactivity. For some of the T cell clones, such as Ob.A12, amino acid identity was required at two TCR contact residues of the MBP peptide, whereas every TCR contact residue of the MBP peptide could be substituted by at least one structurally related amino acid for other T cell clones.

Two of the T cell clones (Ob.1A12 and Ob.2F3) differed only in the CDR3 loops of TCR α and β because they had identical Vα-Jα and Vβ-Jβ rearrangements (Wucherpfennig et al. 1994b). Nevertheless, the clones differed in the level of cross-reactivity because only three of the five microbial peptides identified for clone Ob.1A12 activated the other clone. We examined the basis for the different level of cross-reactivity and found that the clones had a very similar fine specificity for the MBP peptide, except for the P5 position of the peptide (P5 Lys). The microbial peptides that activated clone Ob.1A12 were characterized by conservative or nonconservative changes at P5 (Lys to Arg, Ser, or Pro). In contrast, clone Ob.2F3 was only stimulated by the peptides that had a conservative lysine-to-arginine substitution. The degree of specificity in recognition of the P5 side chain was the key difference between these TCR because the *Haemophilus influenzae /Escherichia coli* peptide stimulated both clones when the P5 position was substituted from serine to arginine (Hausmann et al. 1999a). In the crystal structure of the HLA-DR2-MBP peptide complex, P5 Lys was a prominent, solvent-exposed residue in the center of the DR2/MBP peptide surface (Fig. 1). In the Ob.1A12 TCR structure this peptide side chain is contacted by the outer surface of the CDR3 loop of TCRβ. The two TCRs differ at one of the residues that makes a direct contact to P5 Lys, accounting for the difference in the degree of TCR crossreactivity (Hahn et al., 2005).

Similar findings were made for MHC class I restricted T cell clones that recognize the HTLV-1 Tax (11–19) peptide bound to HLA-A2. The crystal structure of the MHC–peptide-TCR complex has been determined for both of these TCRs (A6 and B7), which demonstrated major differences in the shape and charge of the TCR pocket for the P5 peptide residue (Garboczi et al. 1996; Ding et al. 1998). The B7 TCR was exquisitely specific for P5 tyrosine of Tax (11–19) because only aromatic substitutions were tolerated. In contrast, the A6 TCR was much more degenerate at the P5 position because 10 of 17 analog peptides induced lysis of target cells at low peptide concentrations (Hausmann et al. 1999b). The absolute requirement for an aromatic side chain by the B7 T cell clone could be explained based on the structure of the P5 pocket: The P5 Tyr represented a tight fit for this TCR pocket and a favorable stacking interaction between the aromatic ring of P5 Tyr, and an aromatic residue of the CDR3 loop of the TCR β chain (Y104 β) was observed. In contrast, the A6 TCR had a larger P5 pocket and the P5 Tyr did not interact with an aromatic TCR residue. These data demonstrate that the TCR CDR3 loops can determine the degree of specificity and degeneracy of the central TCR pocket.

Further characterization of the peptide from the EBV DNA polymerase gene demonstrated a second structural mechanism for TCR cross-reactivity. The HLA-DR2 haplotype that confers susceptibility to MS encodes two DRβ chain genes (DRB1*1501 and DRB5*0101), both of which can pair with the nonpolymorphic DRα chain to form functional DR heterodimers (Sone et al. 1985). Both DR molecules are expressed by antigen-presenting cells in subjects with the HLA-DR2 haplotype. The Hy.2E11 clone recognized the MBP peptide bound to DRA, DRB1*1501 molecules, but surprisingly the EBV peptide bound to DRA, DRB5*0101 molecules. Comparison of the two crystal structures demonstrated a striking degree of similarity, in particular for the peptide positions previously shown to be required for TCR recognition (Lang et al. 2002; Wucherpfennig and Strominger 1995). TCR cross-reactivity can therefore involve the recognition of different peptides bound to the same MHC molecule, or recognition of different peptides on other self-MHC molecules.

8
TCR Cross-Reactivity and Immunopathology

Several different experimental autoimmune diseases have been induced by immunization with microbial peptides, indicating that cross-reactive T cell populations can be pathogenic. EAE has been induced in different strains of mice and in Lewis rats with mimicry peptides of MBP and myelin oligodendrocyte glycoprotein (Ufret-Vincenty et al. 1998; Grogan et al. 1999; Gautam et al. 1998; Mokhtarian et al. 1999; Lenz et al. 2001). However, the physiologically more relevant question is whether autoimmune disease can also result from *infection* with pathogens that carry such T cell epitopes. To address this question, Olson et al. (2001) generated recombinant Theiler's viruses in which the candidate sequences were placed into the leader segment of the virus. The first recombinant virus carried the sequence of the PLP (139–151) peptide that is immunodominant in SJL mice, and infection with this virus resulted in the rapid development of central nervous system (CNS) inflammation and vigorous CD4 T cell responses to the PLP peptide. It is important to note that the wild-type Theiler's virus also induced CNS pathology, but disease onset was significantly later (day 30 rather than day 10), permitting the two disease states to be distinguished. Also, tolerance induction with the PLP (139–151) peptide prevented induction of the early disease process with the PLP (139–151)-expressing virus, but not the late disease caused by wild-type Theiler's virus (Olson et al. 2002). Importantly, CNS autoimmunity could be induced not only by a virus that carried the self-peptide, but also by a recombinant virus that expressed a peptide from *Hemophilus influenzae* shown to stimulate PLP (139–151)-specific T cells (Olson et al. 2001).

The relationship between autoimmune disease and viral infection has also been examined with natural pathogens, in particular with the Herpes simplex keratitis (HSK) model (Panoutsakopoulou et al. 2001). Infection of the eye with Herpes simplex virus (HSV-1, KOS strain) triggers a T cell-mediated autoimmune process that persists after the virus has been cleared. To rigorously test the role of molecular mimicry in this disease process, a single amino acid substitution was made in the cross-reactive T cell epitope of the viral UL-6 protein. The mimicry T cell epitope was found to be important for disease induction in C.AL-20 mice because 1,000-fold larger quantities of the mutant virus were required than of wild-type HSV-1, even though both viruses replicated at the same rate. However, in mice that expressed the Cl-6 TCR and therefore harbored large numbers of autoreactive T cells, infection with HSV-1 was not required because scratching of the cornea or local application of LPS was sufficient for the induction of disease. The cross-reactive T cell epitope was thus required for the expansion of autoreactive T cells, but activation of the innate immune system was sufficient when large numbers of such T cells were already present. This model therefore clarified the potential contributions of TCR cross-reactivity and "bystander" activation in the induction of autoimmune diseases.

The diverse nature of the viral/bacterial peptides that stimulate autoreactive T cell clones suggests that different infectious agents could initiate autoimmunity by molecular mimicry. However, it is important to keep in mind that a number of other mechanisms could also result in the activation of autoreactive T cells. The diverse nature of the mimicry peptides and the ubiquitous presence of some of these pathogens may make it difficult to establish a direct epidemiological link between infectious agents and the occurrence of certain autoimmune diseases. In particular, the temporal relationship between an infection and development of an autoimmune process may in many cases not be clear because of the time that frequently elapses before clinical symptoms become obvious and a diagnosis is made. Such epidemiological relationships may be more readily established for autoimmune disorders with a rapid disease onset because early diagnosis can greatly increase the likelihood of establishing a link with a preceding infection. Recent data have demonstrated a relationship between an inflammatory, demyelinating disease of the peripheral nervous system (Guillain-Barré syndrome) and preceding infections (Rees et al. 1995). Patients with this disease acutely develop severe symptoms, and rapid diagnosis permitted isolation of *Campylobacter jejuni* from approximately a third of new cases, compared to 2% of household controls. A better understanding of the epidemiology of infectious agents and autoimmunity could thus help to advance our understanding of the molecular mechanisms that trigger autoimmune diseases.

9
TCR Cross-Reactivity as a General Property of T Cell Recognition

A large number of studies have now demonstrated TCR cross-reactivity for a variety of human and murine T cells (Bhardwaj et al. 1993; Hemmer et al. 1997; Grogan et al. 1999; Evavold et al. 1995; Hagerty and Allen 1995; Loftus et al. 1996; Misko et al. 1999; Brehm et al. 2002). An interesting example is the melanoma/melanocyte-derived peptide MART-1 (res. 27–35) because it demonstrates how cross-reactivity can shape the T cell repertoire. In normal human donors with the HLA-A2 haplotype, T cells specific for this melanocyte peptide were detected at a surprisingly high frequency, and such T cells could be visualized directly ex vivo with HLA-A2/MART-1 tetramers (frequency of ~0.1%). This suggested that these T cells cross-reacted with microbial peptides, and a motif search similar to the one that we had performed for human MBP specific T cell clones yielded 12 peptides that were able to sensitize target cells for lysis. One of these peptides was derived from the glycoprotein C of HSV, and anti-MART effectors lysed cells infected with a recombinant vaccinia virus encoding HSV-1 glycoprotein C (Loftus et al. 1996; Dutoit et al. 2002).

TCR cross-reactivity can also have a profound effect on protective immune responses to viral pathogens in vivo, as shown in a murine model in which CD8 T cells cross-reacted with peptides from two different viruses—lymphocytic choriomeningitis virus (LCMV) and Pichinde virus (PV) (Brehm et al. 2002). LCMV and PV are members of the *Arenaviridae* family, but the two viruses are only distantly related as shown by sequence comparison. Prior infection with either LCMV or PV provided partial protection against the heterologous virus, and LCMV-immune mice showed a 97% reduction in viral titer compared to naïve mice when challenged with PV. CD8 T cells from mice infected with either virus cross-reacted with a nucleoprotein-derived peptide (NP 205–212) from the other virus; these two nucleoprotein peptides shared six of eight residues and differed at positions 5 (Tyr versus Phe) and 8 (Leu versus Met). In LCMV-infected mice the NP 205–212 epitope was subdominant and 3.6% of CD8 T cells responded to this epitope on day 8 after infection. However, CD8 T cells specific for this NP 205–212 peptide became the predominant CD8 T cell population (30% of all CD8 T cells) when mice that had previously encountered PV were infected with LCMV. These experiments demonstrated that TCR cross-reactivity influences the hierarchy of CD8 T cell responses and shapes the pool of memory T cells.

TCR cross-reactivity is also a critical aspect of T cell development in the thymus, and weaker TCR signals are required for positive selection in the thymus compared to activation of mature T cells. Positive selection in the thymus is peptide dependent and is affected by both the density of a particular MHC–peptide complex and the affinity of the TCR for this complex. In thymic organ cultures, positive selection was observed with peptides that represented weak agonists or antagonists for the corresponding mature T cells, or with low densities of the agonist peptide (Jameson et al. 1994; Sebzda et al. 1994; Alam et al. 1996). The creation of transgenic mice that expressed a single MHC–peptide ligand in the thymus provided a striking demonstration of cross-reactive TCR recognition in thymic development (Ignatowicz et al. 1996). In this experiment, a peptide was covalently linked to the N terminus of the MHC class II β chain so that all MHC class II molecules were occupied with this peptide. The total numbers of CD4 T cells in these mice were ~20% compared to wild-type mice, and these CD4 T cells expressed a wide variety of different Vβ segments, indicating that a relatively diverse T cell repertoire could develop in the presence of a single MHC class II–peptide ligand. T cell hybridomas isolated from these mice reacted with peptides that had no primary sequence identity with the selecting peptide (Ignatowicz et al. 1997). These experiments demonstrated that T cells could be activated by peptides that were unrelated in sequence to their selecting peptide.

The examples described above indicate that TCR cross-reactivity is common and represents an important aspect of TCR recognition. The balance between specificity and cross-reactivity is likely to represent a compromise that permits a sufficient number of T cells to recognize a pathogen novel to the individual's immune system. The potentially negative impact of TCR cross-reactivity may be in part balanced by in vivo selection of T cells with high-avidity TCR for the relevant MHC–peptide complexes. It has been postulated that a single TCR can recognize 10^6 different peptide ligands, and this estimate is based on the observation that a subset of T cell clones can be activated by complex peptide mixtures in which only one peptide position is specified (Mason 1998). Although the number of peptide variants that can be recognized may be very large, the number of natural ligands from microbial and self-antigens is likely to be considerably smaller. Nevertheless, a number of different peptides can act as agonists for a given T cell and a considerably larger number of peptide ligands may induce weak signals, such as those that promote positive selection in the thymus and survival of naïve T cells in the periphery. TCR specificity and cross-reactivity thus represent important aspects of T cell biology.

Acknowledgements I would like to acknowledge the important contributions that my colleagues and collaborators have made toward this research. In particular, I would like to acknowledge the contributions of Stefan Hausmann, Katherine Smith, Laurent Gauthier, Heiner Appel, Jason Pyrdol, David A. Hafler, Don C. Wiley, and Jack L. Strominger. This work was supported by grants from the National Multiple Sclerosis Society and the NIH (R01 AI064177 and P01 AI45757).

References

Alam S.M., Travers P.J., Wung J.L., Nasholds W., Redpath S., Jameson S.C., Gascoigne N.R. 1996. T-cell-receptor affinity and thymocyte positive selection. Nature 381, 616–620

Ausubel L.J., Kwan C.K., Sette A., Kuchroo V., Hafler D.A. 1996. Complementary mutations in an antigenic peptide allow for crossreactivity of autoreactive T-cell clones. Proc. Natl. Acad. Sci. U S A 93, 15317–15322

Bhardwaj V., Kumar V., Geysen H.M., Sercarz E.E. 1993. Degenerate recognition of a dissimilar antigenic peptide by myelin basic protein-reactive T cells. Implications for thymic education and autoimmunity. J. Immunol. 151, 5000–5010

Brehm M.A., Pinto A.K., Daniels K.A., Schneck J.P., Welsh R.M., Selin L.K. 2002. T cell immunodominance and maintenance of memory regulated by unexpectedly cross-reactive pathogens. Nat. Immunol. 3, 627–634

Brown J.H., Jardetzky T.S., Gorga J.C., Stern L.J., Urban R.G., Strominger J.L., Wiley D.C. 1993. Three-dimensional structure of the human class II histocompatibility antigen HLA-DR1. Nature 364, 33–39

Burrows S.R., Khanna R., Burrows J.M., Moss D.J. 1994. An alloresponse in humans is dominated by cytotoxic T lymphocytes (CTL) cross-reactive with a single Epstein-Barr virus CTL epitope: implications for graft-versus-host disease. J. Exp. Med. 179, 1155–1161

Chicz R.M., Urban R.G., Gorga J.C., Vignali D.A., Lane W.S., Strominger J.L. 1993. Specificity and promiscuity among naturally processed peptides bound to HLA-DR alleles. J. Exp. Med. 178, 27–47

Datta A.K., Feighny R.J., Pagano J.S. 1980. Induction of Epstein-Barr virus-associated DNA polymerase by 12-O-tetradecanoylphorbol-13-acetate. Purification and characterization. J. Biol. Chem. 255, 5120–5125

Ding Y.H., Smith K.J., Garboczi D.N., Utz U., Biddison W.E., Wiley D.C. 1998. Two human T cell receptors bind in a similar diagonal mode to the HLA- A2/Tax peptide complex using different TCR amino acids. Immunity 8, 403–411

Dutoit V., Rubio-Godoy V., Pittet M.J., Zippelius A., Dietrich P.Y., Legal F.A., Guillaume P., Romero P., Cerottini J.C., Houghten R.A., Pinilla C., Valmori D. 2002. Degeneracy of antigen recognition as the molecular basis for the high frequency of naive A2/Melan-a peptide multimer(+) CD8(+) T cells in humans. J. Exp. Med. 196, 207–216

Evavold B.D., Sloan-Lancaster J., Wilson K.J., Rothbard J.B., Allen P.M. 1995. Specific T cell recognition of minimally homologous peptides: evidence for multiple endogenous ligands. Immunity 2, 655–663

Fujinami R.S., Oldstone M.B. 1985. Amino acid homology between the encephalitogenic site of myelin basic protein and virus: mechanism for autoimmunity. Science 230, 1043–1045

Garboczi D.N., Ghosh P., Utz U., Fan Q.R., Biddison W.E., Wiley D.C. 1996. Structure of the complex between human T-cell receptor, viral peptide and HLA-A2. Nature 384, 134–141

Garcia K.C., Degano M., Pease L.R., Huang M., Peterson P.A., Teyton L., Wilson I.A. 1998. Structural basis of plasticity in T cell receptor recognition of a self peptide-MHC antigen. Science 279, 1166–1172

Gautam A.M., Liblau R., Chelvanayagam G., Steinman L., Boston T. 1998. A viral peptide with limited homology to a self peptide can induce clinical signs of experimental autoimmune encephalomyelitis. J. Immunol. 161, 60–64

Gautam A.M., Lock C.B., Smilek D.E., Pearson C.I., Steinman L., McDevitt H.O. 1994. Minimum structural requirements for peptide presentation by major histocompatibility complex class II molecules: implications in induction of autoimmunity. Proc. Natl. Acad. Sci. U S A 91, 767–771

Grogan J.L., Kramer A., Nogai A., Dong L., Ohde M., Schneider-Mergener J., Kamradt T. 1999. Cross-reactivity of myelin basic protein-specific T cells with multiple microbial peptides: experimental autoimmune encephalomyelitis induction in TCR transgenic mice. J. Immunol. 163, 3764–3770

Hagerty D.T., Allen P.M. 1995. Intramolecular mimicry. Identification and analysis of two cross-reactive T cell epitopes within a single protein. J. Immunol. 155, 2993–3001

Hahn M., Nicholson M. J., Pyrdol J., and Wucherpfennig K.W. 2005. Unconventional topology of self peptide-major histocompatibility complex binding by a human autoimmune T cell receptor. Nat. Immunol 6, 490–496.

Hammer J., Valsasnini P., Tolba K., Bolin D., Higelin J., Takacs B., Sinigaglia F. 1993. Promiscuous and allele-specific anchors in HLA-DR-binding peptides. Cell 74, 197–203

Hausmann S., Biddison W.E., Smith K.J., Ding Y.H., Garboczi D.N., Utz U., Wiley D.C., Wucherpfennig K.W. 1999b. Peptide recognition by two HLA-A2/Tax11–19-specific T cell clones in relationship to their MHC/peptide/TCR crystal structures. J. Immunol. 162, 5389–5397

Hausmann S., Martin M., Gauthier L., Wucherpfennig K.W. 1999a. Structural features of autoreactive TCR that determine the degree of degeneracy in peptide recognition. J. Immunol. 162, 338–344

Hemmer B., Fleckenstein B.T., Vergelli M., Jung G., McFarland H., Martin R., Wiesmuller K.H. 1997. Identification of high potency microbial and self ligands for a human autoreactive class II-restricted T cell clone. J. Exp. Med. 185, 1651–1659

Hennecke J., Carfi A., and Wiley D.C. 2000. Structure of a covalently stabilized complex of a human $\alpha\beta$ T-cell receptor, influenza HA peptide and MHC class II molecule, HLA-DR1. Embo J 19, 5611–5624.

Hunt D.F., Michel H., Dickinson T.A., Shabanowitz J., Cox A.L., Sakaguchi K., Appella E., Grey H.M., Sette A. 1992. Peptides presented to the immune system by the murine class II major histocompatibility complex molecule I-Ad. Science 256, 1817–1820

Ignatowicz L., Kappler J., Marrack P. 1996. The repertoire of T cells shaped by a single MHC/peptide ligand. Cell 84, 521–529

Ignatowicz L., Rees W., Pacholczyk R., Ignatowicz H., Kushnir E., Kappler J., Marrack P. 1997. T cells can be activated by peptides that are unrelated in sequence to their selecting peptide. Immunity 7, 179–186

Jameson S.C., Hogquist K.A., Bevan M.J. 1994. Specificity and flexibility in thymic selection. Nature 369, 750–752

Lang H.L., Jacobsen H., Ikemizu S., Andersson C., Harlos K., Madsen L., Hjorth P., Sondergaard L., Svejgaard A., Wucherpfennig K., Stuart D.I., Bell J.I., Jones E.Y., Fugger L. 2002. A functional and structural basis for TCR cross-reactivity in multiple sclerosis. Nat. Immunol. 3, 940–943

Lenz D.C., Lu L., Conant S.B., Wolf N.A., Gerard H.C., Whittum-Hudson J.A., Hudson A.P., Swanborg R.H. 2001. A *Chlamydia pneumoniae*-specific peptide induces experimental autoimmune encephalomyelitis in rats. J. Immunol. 167, 1803–1808

Loftus D.J., Castelli C., Clay T.M., Squarcina P., Marincola F.M., Nishimura M.I., Parmiani G., Appella E., Rivoltini L. 1996. Identification of epitope mimics recognized by CTL reactive to the melanoma/melanocyte-derived peptide MART-1(27–35). J. Exp. Med. 184, 647–657

Mason D. 1998. A very high level of crossreactivity is an essential feature of the T-cell receptor. Immunol. Today 19, 395–404

Misko I.S., Cross S.M., Khanna R., Elliott S.L., Schmidt C., Pye S.J., Silins S.L. 1999. Crossreactive recognition of viral, self, and bacterial peptide ligands by human class I-restricted cytotoxic T lymphocyte clonotypes: implications for molecular mimicry in autoimmune disease. Proc. Natl. Acad. Sci. U S A 96, 2279–2284

Mokhtarian F., Zhang Z., Shi Y., Gonzales E., Sobel R.A. 1999. Molecular mimicry between a viral peptide and a myelin oligodendrocyte glycoprotein peptide induces autoimmune demyelinating disease in mice. J. Neuroimmunol. 95, 43–54

Olson J.K., Croxford J.L., Calenoff M.A., Dal Canto M.C., Miller S.D. 2001. A virus-induced molecular mimicry model of multiple sclerosis. J. Clin. Invest. 108, 311–318

Olson J.K., Eagar T.N., Miller S.D. 2002. Functional activation of myelin-specific T cells by virus-induced molecular mimicry. J. Immunol. 169, 2719–2726

Panoutsakopoulou V., Sanchirico M.E., Huster K.M., Jansson M., Granucci F., Shim D.J., Wucherpfennig K.W., Cantor H. 2001. Analysis of the relationship between viral infection and autoimmune disease. Immunity 15, 137–147

Reay P.A., Kantor R.M., Davis M.M. 1994. Use of global amino acid replacements to define the requirements for MHC binding and T cell recognition of moth cytochrome c (93–103). J. Immunol. 152, 3946–3957

Rees J.H., Soudain S.E., Gregson N.A., Hughes R.A. 1995. *Campylobacter jejuni* infection and Guillain-Barre syndrome. N. Engl. J. Med. 333, 1374–1379

Sebzda E., Wallace V.A., Mayer J., Yeung R.S., Mak T.W., Ohashi P.S. 1994. Positive and negative thymocyte selection induced by different concentrations of a single peptide. Science 263, 1615–1618

Smith K.J., Pyrdol J., Gauthier L., Wiley D.C., Wucherpfennig K.W. 1998. Crystal structure of HLA-DR2 (DRA*0101, DRB1*1501) complexed with a peptide from human myelin basic protein. J. Exp. Med. 188, 1511–1520

Sone T., Tsukamoto K., Hirayama K., Nishimura Y., Takenouchi T., Aizawa M., Sasazuki T. 1985. Two distinct class II molecules encoded by the genes within HLA-DR subregion of HLA-Dw2 and Dw12 can act as stimulating and restriction molecules. J. Immunol. 135, 1288–1298

Stern L.J., Brown J.H., Jardetzky T.S., Gorga J.C., Urban R.G., Strominger J.L., Wiley D.C. 1994. Crystal structure of the human class II MHC protein HLA-DR1 complexed with an influenza virus peptide. Nature 368, 215–221

Ufret-Vincenty R.L., Quigley L., Tresser N., Pak S.H., Gado A., Hausmann S., Wucherpfennig K.W., Brocke S. 1998. In vivo survival of viral antigen-specific T cells that induce experimental autoimmune encephalomyelitis. J. Exp. Med. 188, 1725–1738

Wucherpfennig K.W., Sette A., Southwood S., Oseroff C., Matsui M., Strominger J.L., Hafler D.A. 1994a. Structural requirements for binding of an immunodominant myelin basic protein peptide to DR2 isotypes and for its recognition by human T cell clones. J. Exp. Med. 179, 279–290

Wucherpfennig K.W., Strominger J.L. 1995. Molecular mimicry in T cell-mediated autoimmunity: viral peptides activate human T cell clones specific for myelin basic protein. Cell 80, 695–705

Wucherpfennig K.W., Zhang J., Witek C., Matsui M., Modabber Y., Ota K., Hafler D.A. 1994b. Clonal expansion and persistence of human T cells specific for an immunodominant myelin basic protein peptide. J. Immunol. 152, 5581–5592

A Virus-Induced Molecular Mimicry Model of Multiple Sclerosis

J. K. Olson · A. M. Ercolini · S. D. Miller (✉)

Department of Microbiology-Immunology and Interdepartmental Immunobiology Center, Northwestern University Feinberg School of Medicine, Chicago, IL, USA
s-d-miller@northwestern.edu

1	Introduction	40
2	Virus-Induced Molecular Mimicry Model of Multiple Sclerosis	42
3	*Haemophilus influenzae* Is a Molecular Mimic of $PLP_{139-151}$	45
4	Multiple Infections with Molecular Mimic-Encoding Pathogens Increase Disease Severity	47
5	Infection of the Target Organ Is Not Required for Autoimmune Disease Induced by Molecular Mimicry	47
6	Model for Molecular Mimicry Induced Autoimmune Demyelinating Disease	48
7	Conclusions and Perspectives	50
References		51

Abstract Multiple sclerosis1 (MS) is an immune-mediated autoimmune demyelinating disease in humans. The initiating event in MS is unknown, but epidemiological evidence suggests that virus infections may be important and one possible mechanism for induction of infection-induced autoimmune disease is molecular mimicry. To test the ability of a virus encoding a self myelin mimic epitope to induce an autoimmune response, we have developed a mouse model wherein the immunodominant myelin epitope $PLP_{139-151}$, or mimics of this epitope, were inserted into a nonpathogenic variant of Theiler's murine encephalomyelitis virus (TMEV). SJL mice infected with TMEV containing $PLP_{139-151}$ or a mimic of $PLP_{139-151}$ expressed by the protease IV protein of *Haemophilus influenzae*, sharing only 6/13 amino acids with the native epitope, developed an early-onset demyelinating disease associated with activation of $CD4^+$ T cells reactive with $PLP_{139-151}$. We have used this molecular mimicry model to further address the requirements for mimic epitope processing and presentation during infection and the requirements for TCR recognition and MHC binding of mimic epitopes. We have also investigated whether molecular mimicry may require multiple infections, with either the mimic-encoding virus or an unrelated virus, to initiate autoimmune disease. Finally, we have asked whether a virus encoding a molecular mimic has to directly infect the target organ to induce autoimmune disease. Overall, this virus-induced molecular mimicry model has provided critical information regarding the mechanisms by which infection-induced molecular mimicry can induce autoimmune diseases.

1
Introduction

Multiple sclerosis (MS) is a human autoimmune demyelinating disease with an unknown origin. However, epidemiological evidence suggests that both genetic and environmental factors play a role in development of the $CD4^+$ T cell-mediated demyelination. There is a higher incidence of MS for people living in areas with moderate to cold climates (northern and central Europe, North America, Australia, New Zealand) than for people living in warmer climates (Asia, Africa). This susceptibility to disease remains with individuals that migrate from high-risk areas to low-risk areas, but only if relocation occurs after the age of 15 years (Kurtzke 1993). These data, along with the fact that MS is not often diagnosed in young children, suggest that risk factors accrue for many years before the onset of MS. Epidemics of MS have been reported in Iceland, the Faroe Islands, and the Shetland-Orkney Islands (Kurtzke 2000; Kurtzke et al. 1993; Kurtzke and Hyllested 1979). Together, these studies provide strong circumstantial evidence that infectious agents, particularly those endogenous to areas of high risk, may play an important role in triggering or propagating MS. Much effort has been put into linking specific viral and bacterial infections with the development of MS. One study claims that antigens derived from human herpesvirus type 6 are found in MS plaques, but not in tissues from patients with other neurological conditions (Challoner et al. 1995). Also, cerebrospinal fluid (CSF) from MS patients has been reported to show higher levels of the intracellular bacteria *Chlamydia pneumoniae* than CSF from patients with other neurological diseases (Sriram et al. 1999). Although other reports have contradicted these results (Derfuss et al. 2001), it is well established that relapses or disease flares in patients diagnosed with the relapsing-remitting form of MS are often associated with exogenous infections, in particular, upper respiratory infections (Edwards et al. 1998; Andersen et al. 1993). In total, over 24 viral agents have been linked to MS (Fujinami 2001; Olson et al. 2001b).

There are several possible mechanisms by which a pathogen can induce autoimmune disease. T cells targeting a persistent pathogen may induce bystander damage to the surrounding tissue and lead to the release of self-antigens; the subsequent generation of autoreactive T cells is known as *epitope spreading* (Miller et al. 1997; Olson et al. 2001b; Vanderlugt and Miller 2002). Alternately, autoreactive T cells may be activated in a nonspecific manner by the cytokines and other inflammatory mediators produced during an infection (*bystander activation*). However, the most widely proposed and studied mechanism is *molecular mimicry*, in which T cells generated against foreign epitopes are also cross-reactive with self-epitopes. Several reports have shown that MS patients have activated T cells specific for epitopes on myelin basic protein (MBP) and other myelin proteins, including proteolipid protein (PLP) and myelin oligodendrocyte glycoprotein (MOG) (Allegretta et al. 1990; Wucherpfennig et al. 1994b; Zhang and Raus 1994; Bielekova et al. 2004). Subsequently, eight pathogen-derived peptides including epitopes from herpes simplex virus, adenovirus, and human papillomavirus, were identified and shown to activate MBP-specific T cell clones derived from MS patients (Wucherpfennig and Strominger 1995). Significantly, these peptides were presented most efficiently by subtypes of MHC class II HLA-DR2 that are associated with susceptibility to MS. Although these findings demonstrate that molecular mimicry is a feasible link between infection and MS, the search continues for more direct evidence of the role of molecular mimicry in inducing human disease.

It was originally thought that a foreign peptide needed to have significant sequence similarity to self-peptide in order to induce an autoreactive response. It is now known that degeneracy in the TCR allows several different peptides to be recognized by the same T cell clone (Wucherpfennig et al. 1995). Likewise, degeneracy in MHC class II binding (Wucherpfennig et al. 1994a) means that a peptide may need only possess a few critical amino acid residues in order to activate a T cell. "Noncritical" residues may also contribute to degeneracy by affecting the overall structure of the peptide, thereby affecting TCR and MHC binding. One group demonstrated that KRN T cells (expressing a single TCR) recognize a self-peptide presented by one MHC class II molecule and a foreign peptide presented by a different MHCII molecule (Basu et al. 2000, 2001). The two peptides only shared sequence similarity at one residue; thus tight regulation is required to inhibit activation of self-reactive T cells in vivo. Similarly, it was recently shown that two distinct peptides with limited conservation of crucial residues can activate a single TCR when presented by two different MHC molecules (Lang et al. 2002). More specifically, although both MBP_{85-99} and $EBV_{627-641}$ bind DRB1*1501 (HLA-DR2b), only MBP_{85-99} activates the TCR on the human MS patient-derived T cell clone Hy.2E11 when presented in the context of this particular MHC molecule, whereas $EBV_{627-641}$ can activate Hy.2E11 when presented by DRB5*0101 (HLA-DR2a). The inability of $EBV_{627-641}$ to activate Hy.2E11 in the context of DRB1*1501 likely results from a shift in the MHC-binding register. Thus cognate recognition is dependent upon the peptide-binding registry of both the TCR and MHC class II (Wucherpfennig et al. 1994a, 1995; Kohm et al. 2003).

2
Virus-Induced Molecular Mimicry Model of Multiple Sclerosis

Theiler's murine encephalomyelitis virus (TMEV) is a natural mouse pathogen that is neurotropic and establishes a persistent infection in the central nervous system (CNS)-resident microglial cell population. The persistent virus infection of the CNS leads to the activation of virus-specific $CD4^+$ T cells and subsequent development of autoimmune demyelinating disease via the process of epitope spreading to myelin antigens, including the proteolipid protein, $PLP_{139-151}$, epitope and other minor determinants (Miller et al. 1997; Vanderlugt and Miller 2002). TMEV-induced demyelinating disease serves as a mouse model for MS, sharing multiple immunological and pathological characteristics with the human disease.

Another mechanism by which autoimmune diseases may arise after virus infection is molecular mimicry. We thus designed a TMEV mouse model of molecular mimicry-induced autoimmune disease (Olson et al. 2001a). We originally developed a recombinant TMEV that had a 23-amino acid deletion in the region encoding the virus leader protein with the insertion of a *Cla*I restriction enzyme coding site (ΔCla-TMEV). ΔCla-TMEV does not persist in the CNS; thus infected mice do not undergo epitope spreading to myelin antigens and do not develop disease. To determine whether the nonpathogenic ΔCla-TMEV could serve as a vector to test the potential of infection-induced molecular mimicry to initiate CNS autoimmunity, we inserted the coding region for immunodominant encephalitogenic myelin antigen, $PLP_{139-151}$, as a 30-amino acid insertion, $PLP_{130-159}$ (Fig. 1) using the *Cla*I restriction site. The the 30-mer rather than the minimal encephalitogenic epitope was used to ensure that disease could only be induced if the T cell determinant was correctly processed from its flanking residues in the context of the virus infection.

Mice infected with PLP-TMEV developed an early-onset severe demyelinating disease (7–10 days after infection) associated with an early encephalitogenic $PLP_{139-151}$-specific $CD4^+$ T cell response (arising 7 days after infection) (Fig. 2A) compared to wild-type TMEV with a late disease onset (30–40 days after infection) and late development (40–50 days after infection) of $PLP_{139-151}$-specific $CD4^+$ T cell responses (Miller et al. 1997). Tolerance to $PLP_{139-151}$ induced by the i.v. injection of $PLP_{139-151}$-coupled splenocytes into

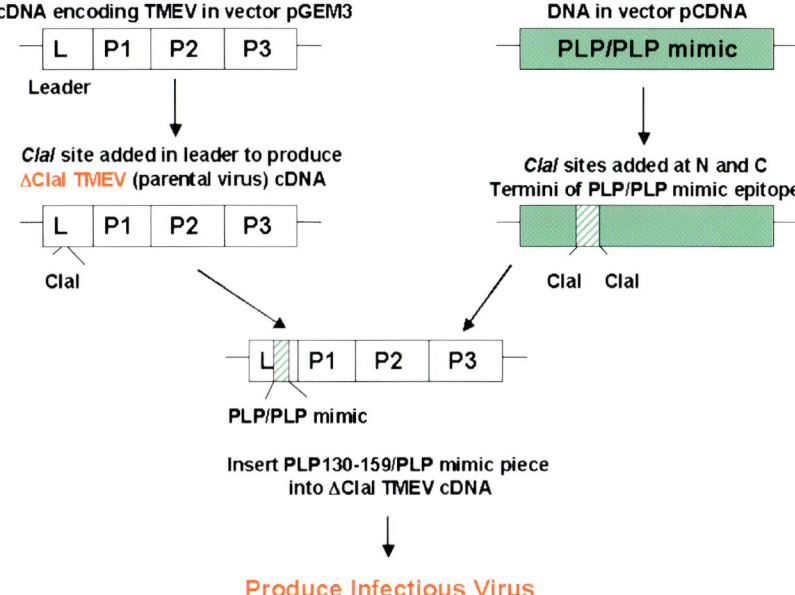

Fig. 1 Construction of TMEV-containing sequences for $PLP_{139-151}$ and molecular mimics of $PLP_{139-151}$. cDNA from TMEV strain BeAn 8386 had a *Cla*I restriction site inserted into the leader sequence, resulting in a 23-amino acid deletion. Amino acid sequences (30–39 residues in length) encompassing the native immunodominant encephalitogenic myelin epitope proteolipid protein epitope, $PLP_{139-151}$, H147A and W144A substituted $PLP_{139-151}$ sequences, a $PLP_{139-151}$ mimic epitope from *H. influenzae*, or $OVA_{323-339}$ control peptide were inserted into the *Cla*I restriction site in the viral cDNA. Viral RNA was synthesized and infectious virus was produced in BHK-21 cells and tested for the ability to induce early-onset demyelinating disease

the mouse before infection with the PLP-TMEV prevented development of demyelinating disease concomitant with reduction of the $PLP_{139-151}$-specific $CD4^+$ T cell response (Olson et al. 2002). In addition, $PLP_{139-151}$-specific $CD4^+$ T cells activated after PLP-TMEV infection were encephalitogenic, as demonstrated by the ability of these cells to induce disease when transferred to naïve recipient mice. These data provide proof of principle that SJL mice infected with TMEV encoding an immunodominant encephalitogenic myelin epitope develop a pathological CNS autoimmune disease due to infection-induced *molecular identity*. Mice infected with ΔCla-TMEV engineered to express the non-self $OVA_{323-339}$ epitope (OVA-TMEV) did not develop the early-onset demyelinating disease (Fig. 2B) but, interestingly, developed late-onset demyelinating disease similar to mice infected with wild-type TMEV.

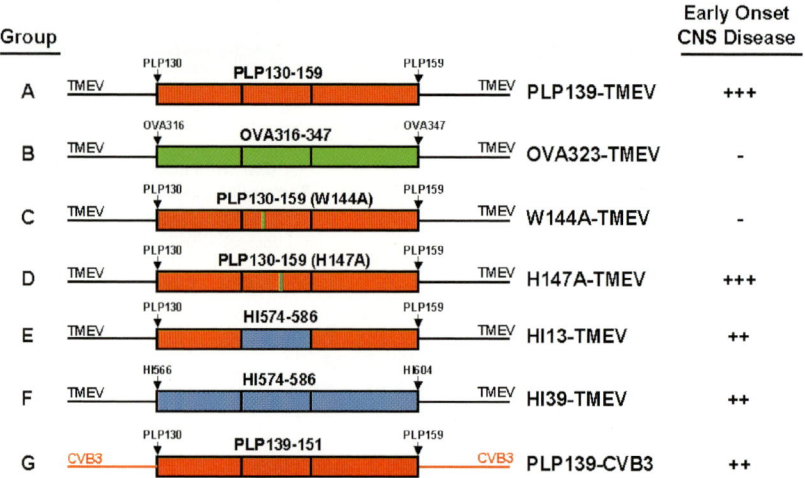

Fig. 2 Summary of induction of early-onset demyelinating disease following intracerebral infection of SJL mice with picornaviruses expressing molecular mimics of $PLP_{139-151}$. Figure shows a pictorial version of the ability of TMEV encoding $PLP_{139-151}$, $OVA_{323-339}$, and various molecular mimics of $PLP_{139-151}$ to induced early-onset demyelinating disease following intracerebral infection of SJL mice

To provide proof of principle for infection-induced molecular mimicry in initiation of CNS autoimmunity, we next engineered the nonpathogenic parental ΔCla-TMEV virus to express mimic $PLP_{139-151}$ sequences containing nonconservative amino acid substitutions in either the primary or secondary T cell receptor (TCR) recognition sites (Olson et al. 2001a). Infection of mice with TMEV containing $PLP_{139-151}$ with a nonconservative substitution in the primary TCR site (residue 144), W144A-TMEV, did not induce an early-onset demyelinating disease and did not activate early cross-reactive $PLP_{139-151}$-specific $CD4^+$ T cell response (Fig. 2C); however, these mice developed the late-onset demyelinating disease similar to the wild-type TMEV-infected mice. In contrast, mice infected with TMEV containing $PLP_{139-151}$ with a conservative substitution at the secondary TCR recognition site (residue 147), H147A-TMEV, developed early-onset demyelinating disease and activated cross-reactive $PLP_{139-151}$-specific $CD4^+$ T cell responses similar to the mice infected with the native PLP-TMEV (Fig. 2D). These mimic viruses demonstrate that a virus encoding an epitope with a similar sequence to self-antigen can induce an autoimmune disease with cross-reactive $CD4^+$ T cell response. These viruses further demonstrate that essential MHC class II and TCR recognition sites must be maintained for the TMEV-encoded mimic epitope to induce CNS autoimmune disease.

3
Haemophilus influenzae Is a Molecular Mimic of PLP$_{139-151}$

Next, we wanted to directly test whether a molecular mimic from a microbe could induce cross-reactive response to PLP$_{139-151}$ and induce demyelinating disease. PLP-TMEV was engineered to express a PLP$_{139-151}$ mimic peptide derived from the protease IV protein (*sppA*) of *Haemophilus influenzae*, HI$_{574-586}$ (HI-TMEV) (Carrizosa et al. 1998). This peptide shares 6 of 13 amino acids with PLP$_{139-151}$ including the primary TCR contact residue at position 144 and the primary and secondary MHC class II binding residues (positions 145 and 148) (Figs. 2E, 3B). HI-TMEV-infected mice developed early-onset demyelinating disease, although the clinical disease was not as severe as that observed in PLP-TMEV-infected mice (Fig. 3B) (Olson et al. 2001a). HI-TMEV disease induction was characterized by the activation of CD4$^+$ IFN-γ-producing Th1 cells responsive to both HI$_{574-586}$ and PLP$_{139-151}$ (Fig. 3C) and by CNS infiltration of activated CD4$^+$ T cells and F4/80$^+$ macrophages/microglia. Further, peripheral tolerance to either PLP$_{139-151}$ or HI$_{574-586}$ before infection with HI-TMEV or PLP-TMEV decreased clinical disease and PLP$_{139-151}$-specific CD4$^+$ T cell responses, definitively proving that the infection-induced disease was due to the cross-activation of autoreactive PLP$_{139-151}$-specific T cells (Croxfort et al. 2005a).

We further wanted to determine whether HI$_{574-586}$ was a natural peptide mimic, i.e., could it be processed and presented from within its native sequence. A 39-amino acid coding region (HI$_{566-604}$) from *H. influenzae* protease IV gene that encompassed the core epitope HI$_{574-586}$ mimic epitope was inserted into the ΔCla-TMEV (HI39-TMEV). Mice infected with HI39-TMEV developed an early-onset demyelinating clinical disease, again not as severe as PLP-TMEV infected mice, but similar to HI-TMEV infected mice (Figs. 2F, 3B). HI39-TMEV-infected mice also developed CD4$^+$ Th1-mediated IFN-γ responses to both HI$_{574-586}$ and PLP$_{139-151}$ (Fig. 3C) of magnitude similar to that in mice infected with HI-TMEV, indicating that the mimic can be processed from its native sequence and induce autoreactive PLP$_{139-151}$-specific CD4$^+$ T cells. Interestingly, immunization of SJL mice with HI$_{574-586}$ peptide emulsified in complete Freund's adjuvant (CFA) does not induce autoimmune demyelination. Although HI$_{574-586}$/CFA-immunized mice develop HI$_{574-586}$-specific CD4$^+$ T cell responses, as well as cross-reactive PLP$_{139-151}$-specific CD4$^+$ T cells, unlike mice infected with either HI-TMEV or HI39-TMEV, the cross-reactive T cells produced low levels of IFNγ (Olson et al. 2001a). This latter result indicates that induction of autoimmune disease via molecular mimicry also requires that the infection promotes the induction of adequate innate immune signals to promote activation of pathologic cross-reactive Th1-type

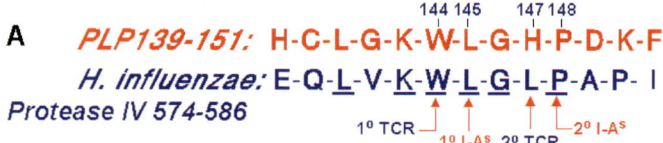
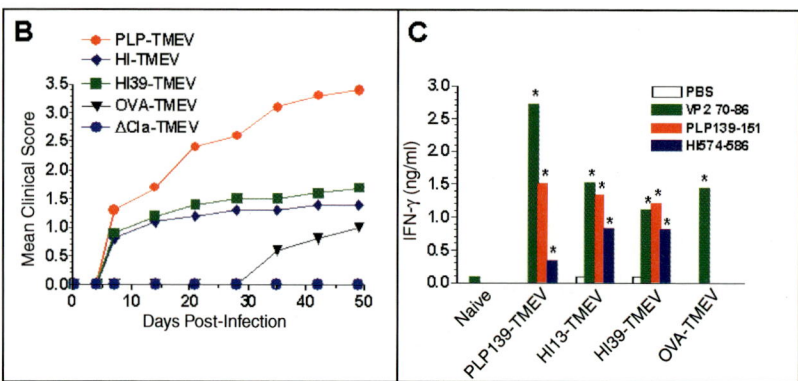

Fig. 3A–C Induction of early-onset demyelinating disease following intracerebral infection of SJL mice with TMEV expressing the native PLP$_{139-151}$ epitope (*PLP-TMEV*) and with a PLP$_{139-151}$ mimic from the protease IV protein of *Haemophilus influenzae* (*HI-TMEV*) is associated with the activation of PLP$_{139-151}$-specific Th1 cells. A Comparison of the amino acid sequence of PLP$_{139-151}$ and the *H. influenzae* protease IV HI$_{574-586}$ molecular mimic indicating the primary and secondary TCR and MHC class II binding residues. B Separate groups of mice (n=8–10) were injected intracerebrally with 3×10^7 PFU of recombinant virus PLP139-TMEV, HI13-TMEV, HI39-TMEV, OVA323-TMEV, or the parental ΔCla-TMEV virus and observed for development of clinical signs of demyelinating disease over a 50-day observation period. C Spleen cells harvested at 21 days PI were rechallenged with viral peptide (*VP2$_{70-86}$*), myelin peptides (*PLP$_{139-151}$*), or mimic peptide (*HI$_{574-586}$*) and supernatants collected after 48 h and measured for IFN-γ secretion by ELISA. *Values significantly above control levels, $p<0.05$

T cell responses. These results indicate that HI$_{574-586}$ can be a naturally processed molecular mimic for PLP$_{139-151}$ only if the proper innate immune stimuli are present during infection. Collectively, these studies definitively indicate that infection of the CNS with a pathogen containing a mimic epitope for a self-myelin antigen can induce a cross-reactive CD4$^+$ T cell response resulting in autoimmune demyelinating disease.

4 Multiple Infections with Molecular Mimic-Encoding Pathogens Increase Disease Severity

As discussed above, epidemiological evidence suggests that MS has a viral etiology based on migration studies, twin studies, and epidemics of MS in Iceland and the Faroe Islands (Kurtzke and Hyllested 1986; Kurtzke et al. 1993; Kurtzke 1997; Sadovnick et al. 1993). One hypothesis based on these studies is that an early childhood infection with a mimic-containing virus may result in an expanded repertoire of autoreactive T cells that may become autoreactive memory T cells. These autoreactive memory T cells may be reactivated on secondary infection with the same virus or a different virus. MS patients often report respiratory infections preceding the onset of MS symptoms (relapses), which would support this hypothesis (Edwards et al. 1998; Andersen et al. 1993).

We have preliminarily investigated the role of secondary infections in the clinical disease severity of mice infected with the $PLP_{139-151}$ mimic-expressing HI-TMEV virus. Mice reinfected with the HI-TMEV virus 14 days after the initial infection developed a severe clinical disease resulting in spastic paralysis and severe inflammation of the CNS (Croxfort et al. 2005b). The second infection with HI-TMEV increased disease severity and inflammation compared to mice infected only once with HI-TMEV. Interestingly, mice infected with HI-TMEV and reinfected with OVA-TMEV also developed a more severe disease, although less severe than the disease in the HI-TMEV-reinfected mice. Therefore, we suggest that after the initial activation of cross-reactive T cells, reinfection with either the primary or a secondary virus can initiate a cascade of events, which leads to an exacerbation of clinical disease. From these results there are numerous possibilities with which to test the hypothesis that molecular mimicry can induce severe autoimmune disease, including reactivation with a secondary infection.

5 Infection of the Target Organ Is Not Required for Autoimmune Disease Induced by Molecular Mimicry

Autoimmune diseases such as MS are organ-specific, with the autoimmune T cell response developing to tissue-specific self-antigens. For molecular mimicry-induced autoimmune disease, it is not known whether the infection must occur primarily in the target organ or whether it can occur in a distal site. Direct infection of the target organ may be important for providing an inflammatory environment for local activation of cross-reactive T cells and may be important for tissue damage to release self-antigens into the inflammatory environment. TMEV is a natural mouse pathogen and is administered by intracerebral injection, resulting in a persistent infection in the CNS throughout the lifetime of the mouse. Thus, in the molecular mimicry-induced TMEV model described above, the virus is injected into the CNS target organ and remains persistent in the CNS (Olson et al. 2001a). To attempt to address the necessity for initial infection of the target organ, we infected SJL mice with PLP-TMEV by various peripheral routes including intraperitoneal, intravenous, and subcutaneous (Olson et al. 2002). Mice infected at peripheral sites developed mild demyelinating disease associated with activation of $PLP_{139-151}$-specific $CD4^+$ T cell responses, suggesting that primary infection outside of the CNS target organ could induce CNS autoimmune disease.

To further determine whether infection of the target organ is necessary for molecular mimicry-induced autoimmune disease, we inserted $PLP_{139-151}$ and $HI_{574-586}$ into Coxsackie virus B3 (CVB3), a related picornavirus that primarily infects the heart and pancreas. Mice infected with $PLP_{130-159}$ expressed in CVB3 (PLP-CVB3) develop an early-onset mild demyelinating disease (Fig. 2G) associated with activation of $PLP_{139-151}$-specific $CD4^+$ T cell response (unpublished results). Thus these results indicate that initial virus infection at a site distal to the eventual target organ of the autoimmune disease can stimulate myelin-reactive CNS-homing T cells via molecular mimicry.

6
Model for Molecular Mimicry Induced Autoimmune Demyelinating Disease

Our current model for virus-induced autoimmune demyelinating disease via molecular mimicry is depicted in Fig. 4. A TMEV encoding a mimic of an encephalitogenic myelin $PLP_{139-151}$ epitope, such as HI-TMEV, infects the CNS and the periphery, which activates $CD4^+$ T cells specific for virus antigens, including the mimic epitope. On infection of the CNS, cytokines and chemokines are expressed that attract $CD4^+$ T cells and professional antigen-presenting cells (APCs) to the CNS and promote the activation of Th1 type T cells. The local antigen-presenting cells, microglia, become activated on infection, upregulate MHC class II and costimulatory molecules, and efficiently present viral antigens to the infiltrating $CD4^+$ T cells (Olson et al. 2001c). Activation of the APCs can result in release of TNF-α and nitric oxide, which have been implicated in directly damaging the myelin surrounding the oligodendrocytes on the axons (Selmaj and Raine 1988; van der Veen et al. 1997). The myelin antigens can then be processed and presented by the activated APCs in

A Virus-Induced Molecular Mimicry Model of Multiple Sclerosis

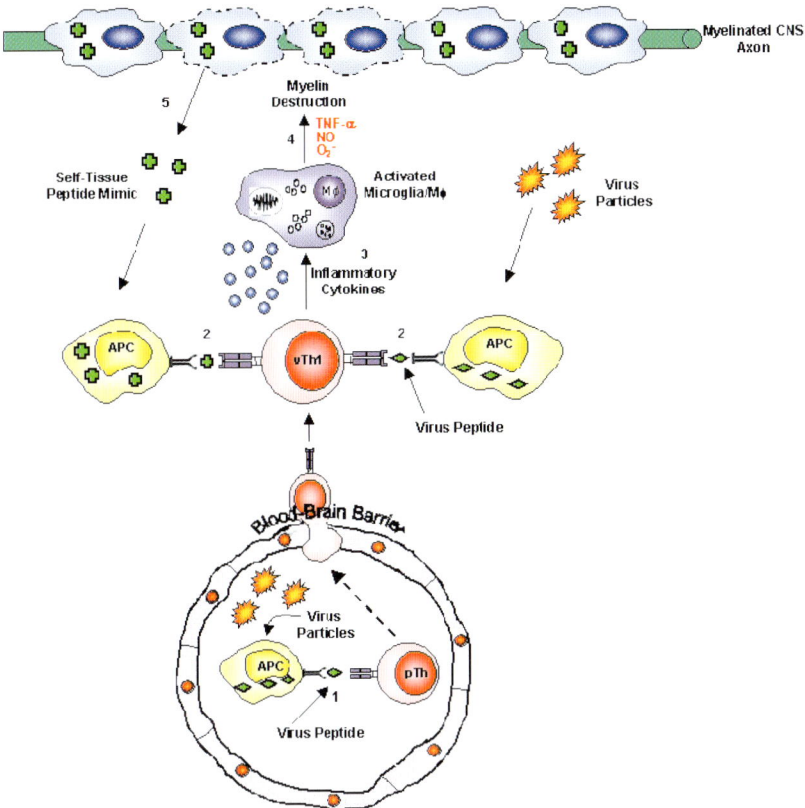

Fig. 4 Molecular mimicry model of autoimmune disease induction. After virus infection, precursor CD4$^+$ precursor T cells are activated by a virus mimic peptide (*1*). Activated virus-specific Th1 (*vTh1*) cells expressing receptors that recognize both the viral epitope and a self-myelin epitope migrate through the blood-brain barrier and enter the CNS parenchyma. Reactivation of the cross-reactive T cells in the infected organ by tissue-resident APCs presenting the self-peptide mimic and the original virus peptide (*2*) results in the release of cytokines and chemokines (*3*) that recruit and activate both tissue-resident and peripheral monocytes/macrophages that mediate myelin damage (*4*). The subsequent release of self-tissue antigens and their uptake and presentation by APCs perpetuates the autoimmune disease (*5*)

the CNS to the mimic epitope-specific CD4$^+$ Th1 cells, which also cross-react with the myelin antigens via molecular mimicry to induce an autoimmune response. Continued damage from the initial infection or a secondary infection leads to further activation of the myelin-specific CD4$^+$ T cells, resulting in the development of chronic autoimmune demyelinating disease.

7
Conclusions and Perspectives

Collectively, these studies present compelling evidence indicating that virus-induced molecular mimicry can *both* induce and enhance a Th1-mediated CNS autoimmune disease model of MS and may have important implications for explaining the initiation and relapse phases of MS pathogenesis. The finding that $PLP_{139-151}$ tolerance significantly inhibits the incidence and severity of disease following HI-TMEV infection and specifically inhibits *both* $HI_{574-587}$- and $PLP_{139-151}$-specific $CD4^+$ T cell responses definitively demonstrates functional activation of pathological cross-reactive $HI_{574-586}$ and $PLP_{139-151}$ $CD4^+$ T cells. The finding that infection with the HI39-TMEV virus induces a similar early-onset demyelinating disease and similar activation of $PLP_{139-151}$-specific $CD4^+$ Th1 cells as is observed after infection with the HI-TMEV virus demonstrates that the HI mimic sequence is a natural epitope that can processed and presented in vivo by SJL APCs to activate $PLP_{139-151}$-specific autoreactive Th1 cells. This is a significant advance over past descriptions of pathological mimic epitopes, which uniformly employ minimal mimic sequences identified in T cell hybridoma screens for their disease-inducing ability and do not take into account the possibility that the mimic peptide may not be capable of being processed from its surrounding amino acid residues in the native mimic protein. In addition, the model illustrates that a critical component required for infection-induced initiation of autoimmune disease via molecular mimicry is the ability of the pathogen to trigger an appropriate innate immune response leading to efficient expansion and differentiation of pathological autoreactive Th1 responses. Finally, the demonstration that a secondary infection with a myelin mimic-expressing neurotropic virus can exacerbate a mild preexisting CNS disease indicates that mimicry may also trigger clinical relapses in autoimmune disease.

There are numerous outstanding questions relating to molecular mimicry and MS that we hope to address with our mouse model. The potential requirement for target organ infection and persistence of the pathogen in initiation of autoimmune disease by infection-induced molecular mimicry require further study. It is uncertain how similar to the autoepitope a molecular mimic has to be in order to induce disease in the context of infection-induced innate immune signals. In addition to the HI mimic, additional pathogen-derived mimics of $PLP_{139-151}$ have been identified (Carrizosa et al. 1998). These mimics are naturally expressed by a variety of infectious agents including *Escherichia coli*, *Salmonella*, *Candida albicans*, and mouse hepatitis virus. Each mimic varies in the degree of similarity to $PLP_{139-151}$, most significantly at key MHC binding and TCR recognition residues. Viruses containing these mimic sequences are being tested to determine whether these mimics can induce a cross-reactive $PLP_{139-151}$-specific $CD4^+$ T cell response. Another question is, What is the phenotype of the T cell population induced on mimic infection? As discussed here, HI-TMEV-infected mice develop a less severe disease than PLP-TMEV-infected mice. This may suggest that the induced T cell repertoires are different. Studies are under way to determine whether HI-specific $CD4^+$ T cells are a separate population with a few overlaps with the $PLP_{139-151}$-specific $CD4^+$ T cell population, or whether they are a subset within the $PLP_{139-151}$-specific $CD4^+$ T cell population. Another line of investigation is testing whether infection of SJL mice with *H. influenzae* can directly activate autoreactive $PLP_{139-151}$-specific T cells and possibly clinical CNS disease via molecular mimicry. Finally, double transgenic mice expressing a human MBP_{85-99}-specific TCR and either HLA-DR2a or HLA-DR2b are being tested for induction of CNS demyelinating disease after infection with TMEV expressing relevant MBP_{85-99} molecular mimics (Wucherpfennig and Strominger 1995), which may be more relevant to the etiology of human MS.

References

Allegretta, M, Nicklas, JA, Sriram, S, and Albertini, RJ (1990) T cells responsive to myelin basic protein in patients with multiple sclerosis. Science 247:718–721

Andersen, O, Lygner, PE, Bergstrom, T, Andersson, M, and Vahlne, A (1993) Viral infections trigger multiple sclerosis relapses: a prospective seroepidemiological study. J. Neurol. 240:417–422

Basu, D, Horvath, S, Matsumoto, I, Fremont, DH, and Allen, PM (2000) Molecular basis for recognition of an arthritic peptide and a foreign epitope on distinct MHC molecules by a single TCR. J. Immunol. 164:5788–5796

Basu, D, Horvath, S, O'Mara, L, Donermeyer, D, and Allen, PM (2001) Two MHC surface amino acid differences distinguish foreign peptide recognition from autoantigen specificity. J. Immunol. 166:4005–4011

Bielekova, B, Sung, MH, Kadom, N, Simon, R, McFarland, H, and Martin, R (2004) Expansion and functional relevance of high-avidity myelin-specific CD4+ T cells in multiple sclerosis. J. Immunol. 172:3893–3904

Carrizosa, AM, Nicholson, LB, Farzan, M, Southwood, S, Sette, A, Sobel, RA, and Kuchroo, VK (1998) Expansion by self antigen is necessary for the induction of experimental autoimmune encephalomyelitis by T cells primed with a cross-reactive environmental antigen. J. Immunol. 161:3307–3314

Challoner, PB, Smith, KT, Parker, JD, MacLeod, DL, Coulter, SN, Rose, TM, Shultz, ER, Bennett, JL, Garber, RL, Chang, M, Schad, PA, Stewart, PM, Nowinski, RC, Brown, JP, and Burmer, GC (1995) Plaque-associated expression of human herpesvirus 6 in multiple sclerosis. Proc. Natl. Acad. Sci. USA 92:7440–7444

Croxford, JL, Anger, HA, and Miller, SD (2005) Viral delivery of an epitope from Haemophilus influenzae induces central nervous system autoimmune disease by molecular mimicry. J. Immunol. 174:907–917

Croxford, JL, Olson, JK, Anger, HA, and Miller, SD (2005) Initiation and exacerbation of CNS autoimmune demyelination via virus-induced molecular mimicry: implications for MS pathogenesis. J. Virol. 79:8581–8590

Derfuss, T, Gurkov, R, Then, BF, Goebels, N, Hartmann, M, Barz, C, Wilske, B, Autenrieth, I, Wick, M, Hohlfeld, R, and Meinl, E (2001) Intrathecal antibody production against *Chlamydia pneumoniae* in multiple sclerosis is part of a polyspecific immune response. Brain 124:1325–1335

Edwards, S, Zvartau, M, Clarke, H, Irving, W, and Blumhardt, LD (1998) Clinical relapses and disease activity on magnetic resonance imaging associated with viral upper respiratory tract infections in multiple sclerosis. J. Neurol. Neurosurg. Psychiatry 64:736–741

Fujinami, RS (2001) Can virus infections trigger autoimmune disease? J. Autoimmun. 16:229–234

Kohm, AP, Fuller, KG, and Miller, SD (2003) Mimicking the way to autoimmunity: an evolving theory of sequence and structural homology. Trends Microbiol. 11:101–105

Kurtzke, JF (1997). The epidemiology of multiple sclerosis. In Multiple Sclerosis: Clinical and Pathogenetic basis. Raine, CS, McFarlin, HF, and Tourtellotte, WW, eds. (London: Chapman and Hall), pp. 91–139.

Kurtzke, JF (1993) Epidemiologic evidence for multiple sclerosis as an infection. Clin. Microbiol. Rev. 6:382–427

Kurtzke, JF (2000) Multiple sclerosis in time and space–geographic clues to cause. J. Neurovirol. 6 Suppl. 2: S134-S140

Kurtzke, JF, Gudmundsson, KR, and Bergmann, S (1993) Multiple sclerosis in Iceland. I. Evidence of a postwar epidemic. Neurology 32:143–150

Kurtzke, JF and Hyllested, K (1979) Multiple sclerosis in the Faroe Islands. I. Clinical and epidemiological features. Ann. Neurol. 5:6-21

Kurtzke, JF and Hyllested, K (1986) Multiple sclerosis in the Faroe Islands. II. Clinical update, transmission, and the nature of MS. Neurology 36:307–328

Lang, HL, Jacobsen, H, Ikemizu, S, Andersson, C, Harlos, K, Madsen, L, Hjorth, P, Sondergaard, L, Svejgaard, A, Wucherpfennig, K, Stuart, DI, Bell, JI, Jones, EY, and Fugger, L (2002) A functional and structural basis for TCR cross-reactivity in multiple sclerosis. Nat. Immunol. 3:940–943

Miller, SD, Vanderlugt, CL, Begolka, WS, Pao, W, Yauch, RL, Neville, KL, Katz-Levy, Y, Carrizosa, A, and Kim, BS (1997) Persistent infection with Theiler's virus leads to CNS autoimmunity via epitope spreading. Nat. Med. 3:1133–1136

Olson, JK, Croxford, JL, Calenoff, M, Dal Canto, MC, and Miller, SD (2001a) A virus-induced molecular mimicry model of multiple sclerosis. J. Clin. Invest. 108:311–318

Olson, JK, Croxford, JL, and Miller, SD (2001b) Virus-induced autoimmunity: Potential role of viruses in initiation, perpetuation, and progression of T cell-mediated autoimmune diseases. Viral Immunol. 14:227–250

Olson, JK, Eagar, TN, and Miller, SD (2002) Functional activation of myelin-specific T cells by virus-induced molecular mimicry. J. Immunol. 169:2719–2726

Olson, JK, Girvin, AM, and Miller, SD (2001c) Direct activation of innate and antigen presenting functions of microglia following infection with Theiler's virus. J. Virol. 75:9780–9789

Sadovnick, AD, Armstrong, H, Rice, GP, Bulman, D, Hashimoto, L, Paty, DW, Hashimoto, SA, Warren, S, Hader, W, and Murray, TJ (1993) A population-based study of multiple sclerosis in twins: update. Ann. Neurol. 33:281–285

Selmaj, K and Raine, CS (1988) Tumor necrosis factor mediates myelin and oligodendrocyte damage in vitro. Ann. Neurol. 23:339–346

Sriram, S, Stratton, CW, Yao, S, Tharp, A, Ding, L, Bannan, JD, and Mitchell, WM (1999) *Chlamydia pneumoniae* infection of the central nervous system in multiple sclerosis. Ann. Neurol. 46:6-14

Vanderlugt, CL and Miller, SD (2002) Epitope spreading in immune-mediated diseases: implications for immunotherapy. Nat. Rev. Immunol. 2:85–95

van der Veen, RC, Hinton, DR, Incardonna, F, and Hofman, FM (1997) Extensive peroxynitrite activity during progressive stages of central nervous system inflammation. J. Neuroimmunol. 77:1-7

Wucherpfennig, KW, Hafler, DA, and Strominger, JL (1995) Structure of human T-cell receptors specific for an immunodominant myelin basic protein peptide: positioning of T-cell receptors on HLA-DR2/peptide complexes. Proc. Natl. Acad. Sci. USA 92:8896–8900

Wucherpfennig, KW, Sette, A, Southwood, S, Oseroff, C, Matsui, M, Strominger, JL, and Hafler, DA (1994a) Structural requirements for binding of an immunodominant myelin basic protein peptide to DR2 isotypes and for its recognition by human T cell clones. J. Exp. Med. 179: 279–290

Wucherpfennig, KW and Strominger, JL (1995) Molecular mimicry in T cell-mediated autoimmunity: viral peptides activate human T cell clones specific for myelin basic protein. Cell 80:695–705

Wucherpfennig, KW, Zhang, J, Witek, C, Matsui, M, Modabber, Y, Ota, K, and Hafler, D (1994b) Clonal expansion and persistence of human T cells specific for an immunodominant myelin basic protein peptide. J. Immunol. 152:5581–5592

Zhang, J and Raus, J (1994) Myelin basic protein-reactive T cells in multiple sclerosis: pathologic relevance and therapeutic targeting. Cytotechnology 16:181–187

Suppression of Autoimmunity via Microbial Mimics of Altered Peptide Ligands

L. Steinman[1] (✉) · P. J. Utz[2] · W. H. Robinson[2]

[1]Dept. of Neurological Sciences and Interdepartmental Program in Immunology, Beckman Center for Molecular Medicine B002, Stanford University School of Medicine, Stanford, CA 94305, USA
steinman@stanford.edu

[2]Division of Immunology and Rheumatology, Department of Medicine, Stanford University School of Medicine, Stanford, CA 94305, USA

1	Microbial Mimics Resembling Altered Peptide Ligands Modulate Animal Models of MS	56
2	Viral Damage, Subsequent Breakdown in Self-Tolerance, and Epitope Spreading In Animal Models of MS	57
References		61

Abstract Molecular mimics of self-antigens can behave as altered peptide ligands and serve to ameliorate autoimmune disease. Analysis of experimental autoimmune encephalomyelitis with proteomic autoantibody microarrays reveals that there might exist a wide variety of microbes with features that mimic self-epitopes. Autoimmunity could therefore be modulated via microbial immunity, which may account for relapse and remission of ongoing disease.

Fujinami and Oldstone demonstrated molecular mimicry between myelin basic protein (MBP) and hepatitis B (Hep B) viral polymerase. When a common stretch of six amino acids shared between MBP and HepB polymerase was injected into rabbits, the animals developed inflammatory brain lesions characteristic of experimental autoimmune encephalomyelitis (EAE) (Fujinami and Oldstone 1985). This seminal paper provided the foundation for the idea that structural mimicry between microbes and self could lead to autoimmunity, when an immune response launched during an infection with a microbe cross-reacts with self.

Molecular mimicry refers to structural homologies between a self-protein and a microbial protein. The concept of molecular mimicry might have pathological consequences and provide a basis for the relapses and remissions so often characteristic of autoimmune disease. For example, molecular mimics may actually modulate the course of multiple sclerosis (MS) and other autoimmune diseases. Consider these examples, based on the immune response in humans with MS to an epitope of MBP: A major epitope of MBP, p87–99 (VHFFKNIVTPRTP), induces EAE in rats and in mice and is a major target of the immune response in MS (Sakai et al. 1988; Bielekova et al. 2000; Kappos et al. 2000; Steinman 2001, 2004). Intravenous tolerization to the MBPp87–99 epitope in patients with MS leads to the abrogation of anti-MBP antibodies, an effect lasting for months after a single intravenous injection (Warren et al. 1997). In a placebo-controlled double-blinded study administration of an altered peptide ligand (APL) of MBPp87–99 reduced the number of active lesions enhancing with gadolinium on magnetic resonance scans (Kappos et al. 2000). These two examples from actual clinical trials with MS patients emphasize how an immune response to MBPp87–99 or to an APL based on MBPp87–99 can either provoke disease or tolerize during the course of ongoing disease. These clinical examples point to the potential relevance of the "molecular mimicry" hypothesis when applied to human disease.

1
Microbial Mimics Resembling Altered Peptide Ligands Modulate Animal Models of MS

The pentapeptide VHFFK contains the major residues for binding of this self-molecule to the TCR receptor (TCR), to the human leukocyte antigen DR2 molecule of the major histocompatibility complex, and to anti-MBP antibodies from MS patients (Warren et al. 1995; Wucherpfennig et al. 1997; Smith et al. 1998). Peptides from papillomavirus strains containing the motif VHFFK induce T cells that are capable of transferring EAE (Ufret-Vincenty et al. 1998). In contrast, Ruiz et al. showed that APL peptides resembling MBPp87–99 peptide, but differing in certain key residues from the native VHFFK, suppressed EAE. Thus a peptide from human papillomavirus type 40 (HPV 40) containing VHFFR, and one from HPV 32 containing VHFFH, prevented EAE (Ruiz et al. 1999). The K residue was shown to be the major TCR contact site in SJL mice for MBPp87–99 (Brocke et al. 1996). Likewise, K at position 91 is the major TCR contact site in humans for T cell clones recognizing the native VHFFK bound to human leukocyte antigen DR2 (Vergelli et al. 1998; Smith et al. 1998).

In our EAE studies, in addition to the sequences from HPV 32 and HPV 40, a sequence from *Bacillus subtilis* (RKVVTDFFKNIPQRI) also prevented EAE. We also showed that T cell lines, producing interleukin 4 and specific for these microbial peptides including HPV40, HPV32, and *Bacillus subtilis*, suppressed EAE, probably by inducing a Th1→Th2 shift (Ruiz et al. 1999).

These findings demonstrated that microbial peptides, differing from the core motif of the self-antigen, MBPp87–99, functioned as altered peptide ligands, and behaved as TCR antagonists, in the modulation of autoimmune disease.

2
Viral Damage, Subsequent Breakdown in Self-Tolerance, and Epitope Spreading In Animal Models of MS

When certain neurotropic viruses trigger inflammation in the central nervous system (CNS), immune cells in the inflammatory infiltrate attack neighboring myelin antigens in the CNS (Miller et al. 1997; Steinman and Conlon 1997). This immune response then spreads to various epitopes on various myelin antigens, a process known as epitope spreading (Lehnmann et al. 1992; Miller et al. 1997). In the context of epitope spreading, molecular mimicry can either exacerbate or ameliorate disease. A virus that mimics one or more of these epitopes that are targeted by the immune system after epitope spreading may trigger a flare-up of demyelinating disease (Ufret-Vincenty et al. 1998),

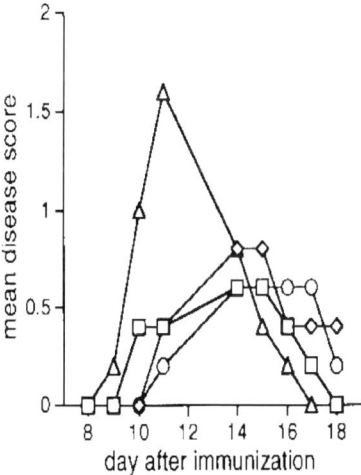

Fig. 1 Prevention of EAE by passive transfer of T cell lines specific for microbial mimicry peptides. Mice were injected intraperitoneally with 5 (*circles*) transfer, mice were challenged for EAE by immunization with gpSCH. Results are expressed as mean disease score in groups of five animals. From Ruiz PJ, Garren H, Hirschberg DL, Langer-Gould AM, Levite M, Karpuj MV, Southwood S, Sette A, Conlon P, Steinman L (1999) Microbial epitopes act altered eptide ligands to prevent EAE. J Exp Med 189:1275–1284

whereas APLs resembling the immunogenic portion of certain neurotropic viruses can suppress EAE (Ruiz et al. 1999, Fig. 1). Earlier work from my laboratory showed that administration of such APLs could lead to the widespread clearance of inflammatory infiltrates in the brain. Such infiltrates are comprised of a diverse collection of T cells and B cells in the brain (Brocke et al. 1996). An APL of MBP p87–99 was able to actually cause such a collection to disperse from areas of inflammation.

In EAE and MS we have constructed large-scale proteomic microarrays to assess the diversity of epitope spreading in the autoantibody response (Robinson et al, 2003). The 2,304-feature myelin proteome arrays contain 232 distinct antigens, including proteins and sets of overlapping peptides representing MBP, proteolipid protein, MOG, myelin-associated oligodendrocytic basic protein (MBOP), oligodendrocyte-specific protein (OSP), B-crystallin, cyclic nucleotide phosphodiesterase (CNPase) and Golli-MBP. These arrays

Fig. 2a–c **a** Hierarchical clustering of antigen features with statistically significant differences in myelin proteome array reactivity between sera derived from groups of normal control mice and from groups of mice on recovery from acute EAE induced with PLP(139–151) (day 17), MBP(85–99) (day 22), or spiral cord homogenale (day 25). Mice were later scored daily for 10 weeks to determine the number of relapses for each mouse (indicated in *parentheses*). The average relapse rates for mice included in the primary subnodes of the dendrogram, and *P* values by Mann-Whitney test for the differences in relapse rate between these nodes, are indicated. **b, c** Antigen features with statistically significant differences in array reactivity between subsets of mice with the greatest (three and four) and least (one) number of relapses within groups induced for EAE with PLP(139–151) or MBP(85–99). SAM (Robinson et al. 2003) was used to identify antigen features with statistically significant differences in array reactivity between groups of mice. A hierarchical cluster algorithm based on a pairwise similarity function was applied to order mice based on similarities in their array reactivities for the SAM-identified features (dendrograms depicting cluster relationships are displayed *above* the individual mice), and to order antigen features based on similarities in reactivities in the mice studied (dendrograms displayed to the *right*). Relationships between mice or antigen features are represented by tree dendrograms whose branch lengths reflect the degree of similarity in array reactivity determined by the hierarchical cluster algorithm. After clustering, labels were added above the dendrograms to indicate the location of clusters of mice induced for EAE with different encephalitogens. With permission from Nature Biotechnology, Vol. 21, pp. 1033 to 1039, Protein microarrays guide tolerizing DNA vaccine treatment of autoimmune encephalomyelitis. by Robinson, WH, Fontoura P, Lee BJ, Neuman de Vegvar HE, TomJ, Pedotti R, DiGennaro C, Mitchell DJ, Fong D, Ho PK, Ruiz P, Maverakis E, Stevens D, Bernard CCA, Olsson T, Martin R, Kuchroo VK, van Noort JM, Genain CP, Utz PJ, Garren H, Steinman L, et al.

Suppression of Autoimmunity via Microbial Mimics of Altered Peptide Ligands   59

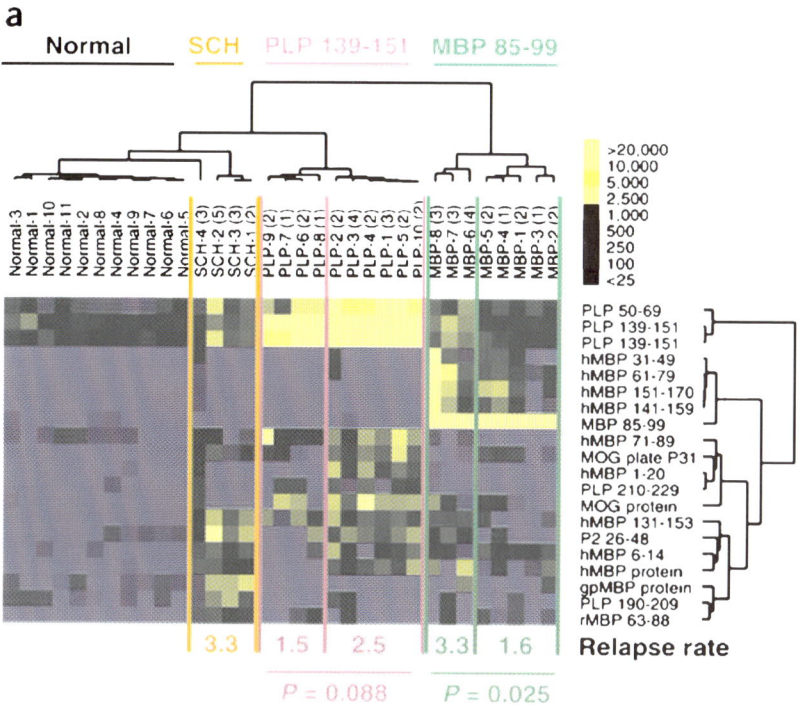

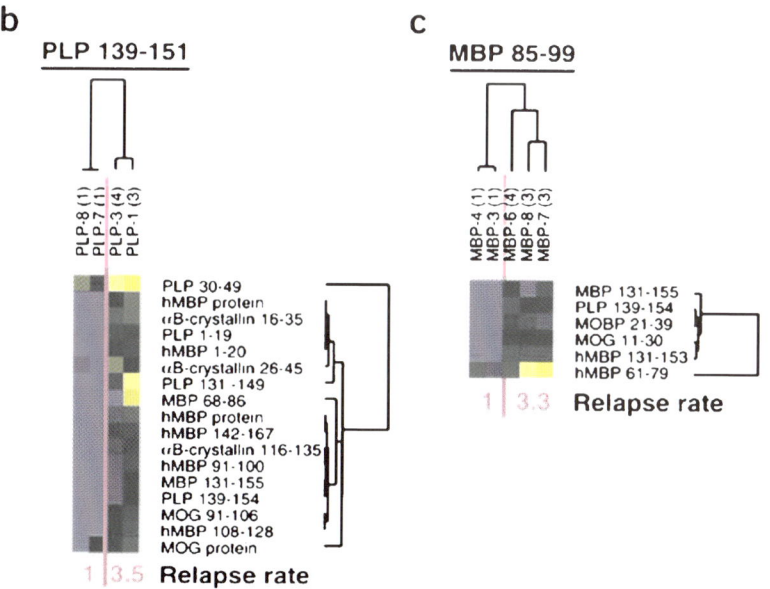

contained 13 proteins and 219 synthetic peptides, including 4 proteins and 85 peptides from MBP, 3 proteins and 30 peptides from PLP, 3 proteins and 50 peptides from MOG, 2 peptides from MBOP, 1 protein and 16 peptides from B-crystallin, 20 peptides from CNPase, 1 protein and 11 peptides from peripheral myelin protein 2 (P2), 2 peptides from the acetylcholine receptor, and 4 nonmyelin peptides or proteins.

We used myelin proteome arrays to profile autoantibody responses in serum derived from mice with EAE, and images of representative arrays are presented in Fig. 2. A similar broad diversity of autoantibody responses is being detected in cerebrospinal fluid of MS patients and in the serum of patients with acute disseminated encephalomyelitis (Robinson et al., in preparation). These studies imply that there might exist a wide variety of microbes with features similar enough to some or even many of these myelin epitopes. If so, then modulation of autoimmunity might be triggered or modulated, similar to what was seen in animal studies of EAE (Wucherpfennig and Strominger 1995; Ufret-Vincenty et al. 1998). A search of the literature reveals that there are a reasonable number of microbes whose structures resemble many of the myelin epitopes that are targeted in EAE (Robinson et al. 2003), and in MS and acute disseminated encephalomyelitis (Robinson et al., in preparation).

First of all it is worth remembering that the homologies between a microbe and its mimic do not have to be extensive. We demonstrated that a polyalanine peptide with only five native MBP residues is able to induce EAE in (PLSJL/J)F1 mice (Gautam et al. 1995) Further analysis also showed that an 11-amino acid peptide, consisting mostly of alanines with only four native Ac1-11 residues, was able to induce T cell hybridoma proliferation. Taking the approach of introducing either D-amino acids or unnatural amino acids in place of L-amino acids into MBPpAc1-11 analogs, we showed that T cells recognize only a short stretch of six or seven amino acids. More importantly, this stretch contains only four native MBPpAc1-11 residues. We also tested T cell recognition in vivo, using EAE as a measure of activation. We showed that a short peptide of six amino acids with a core of only five native Ac1-11 amino acids induces EAE (Karin et al. 1998).

Molecular mimicry between Semliki Forest virus and MOG was shown to induce a chronic onset late EAE, with unusual characteristics including CNS vacuolation. (Mokhtarian et al. 1999). Hughes and coworkers showed that "antisera against MBP (residues 110-124) reacted with both *Acinetobacter* and *Pseudomonas* peptides from 4- and gamma-carboxymuconolactone decarboxylase, respectively. MOG (residues 43-57) antisera reacted with *Acinetobacter* peptide from 3-oxo-adipate-CoA-transferase subunit A" (Hughes et al. 2003). Linington and coworkers have shown interesting homologies between two immunoglobulin supergene family members, MOG and the milk protein butyrophilin (Guggenmos et al. 2004). Zhang and coworkers showed that "greater than 50% of T cells recognizing MBP(93–105) cross-reacted with and could be activated by a synthetic peptide corresponding to residues 1 to 13 of human herpes virus 6 U24 in MS patients" Tejada-Simon et al, 2003].

As we wrote in 1999, "the interaction of the immune system with microbes may allow the selection of viral and bacterial subtypes" (Ruiz et al. 1999). It is interesting to speculate, from our studies with HPV subtypes, "that attenuation of the immune response by a peptide derived from a papilloma viral subtype, containing an APL-like motif, may be desirable for viral survival. A virus capable of subverting the immune response against itself might be selected because it could survive and persist, instead of being eradicated in the wake of an autoimmune response." Arguing from the precedent of T cells specific for MBPp87–99, "there may be a delicate physiological interplay between self- and microbial antigens, allowing the modulation of autoimmune disease and the persistence and survival of mutant microbes. Attenuating inflammation in the brain may allow microbes to survive, sequestered within the central nervous system. It is remarkable that certain viral subtypes are mutated exactly at a main TCR contact site, and such mutations may represent an adaptive response of a virus, which then acts as an APL" (Ruiz et al. 1999). There are now numerous other examples of potential APL-like sequences in other microbial mimics for other epitopes that are targeted by immunity as epitope spreading involves in the course of demyelinating disease (Robinson et al. 2003).

Acknowledgements This work was supported by grants from the National Institutes of Health, the National Multiple Sclerosis Society, and the Phil N. Allen Trust.

References

Bielekova B, Goodwin B, Richert N, Cortese I, Kondo T, Afshar G, Gran B, Eaton J, Antel J, Frank JA, McFarland HF, Martin R (2000) Encephalitogenic potential of the myelin basic protein peptide (amino acids 83–99) in multiple sclerosis: results of a phase II clinical trial with an altered peptide ligand. Nat Med 6(10):1167–1175

Brocke S, Gijbels K, Allegretta M, Ferber I, Piercy C, Blankenstein T, Martin R, Utz U, Karin N, Mitchell D, Veromaa T, Waisman A, Gaur A, Conlon P, Ling N, Fairchild PJ, Wraith DC, O'Garra A, Fathman CG, Steinman L (1996) Treatment of experimental encephalomyelitis with a peptide analogue of myelin basic protein. Nature 379:343–345

Fujinami RS, Olstone MBA (1985) Amino acid homology between the encephalitogenic site of myelin basic protein and virus: mechanism for autoimmunity. Science 230(4729):1043–1045

Gautam AM, Liblau R, Chelvanayagam G, Steinman L, Boston T (1998) A viral peptide with limited homology to a self-peptide can induce clinical signs of experimental autoimmune encephalomyelitis. J Immunol 161:60–64

Guggenmos J, Schubart AS, Ogg S, Andersson M, Olsson T, Mather IH, Linington C (2004) Antibody cross-reactivity between myelin oligodendrocyte glycoprotein and the milk protein butyrophilin in multiple sclerosis. J Immunol 172(1):661–668

Hughes LE, Smith PA, Bonell S, Natt RS, Wilson C, Rashid T, Amor S, Thompson EJ, Croker J, Ebringer A (2003) Cross-reactivity between related sequences found in *Acinetobacter sp.*, *Pseudomonas aeruginosa*, myelin basic protein and myelin oligodendrocyte glycoprotein in multiple sclerosis. J Neuroimmunol 144(1–2):105–115

Kappos L, Comi G, Panitch H, Oger J, Antel J, Conlon P, Steinman L and the APL in Relapsing MS Study Group (2000) Induction of a non-encephalitogenic Th2 autoimmune response in multiple sclerosis after administration of an altered peptide ligand in a placebo controlled, randomized phase II trial. Nat Med 6(10):1176–1182

Karin N, Binah O, Grabie N, Mitchell D, Felzen B, Solomon M, Conlon P, Gaur A, Ling N, Steinman L (1998) Short peptide-based tolerogens without self-antigenic or pathogenic activity reverse autoimmune disease. J Immunol 160:5188–5194

Lehmann P, Forsthuber T, Miller A, Sercarz EE (1992) Spreading of T cell autoimmunity to cryptic determinants of an autoantigen. Nature 358:155–157

Miller SD, Vanderblugt CL, Begolks WS, Pao W, Yauch RL, Neville KL, Katz-Levy Y, Carrizosa A, Kim BS (1997) Persistent infection with Theiler's virus leads to CNS autoimmunity via epitope spreading. Nat Med 3:1133–1136

Mokhtarian F, Zhang Z, Shi Y, Gonzales E, Sobel RA (1999) Molecular mimicry between a viral peptide and a myelin oligodendrocyte glycoprotein peptide induces autoimmune demyelinating disease in mice. J Neuroimmunol 95(1–2):43–54

Robinson, WH, Fontoura P, Lee BJ, Neuman de Vegvar HE, Tom J, Pedotti R, DiGennaro C, Mitchell DJ, Fong D, Ho PK, Ruiz P, Maverakis E, Stevens D, Bernard CCA, Olsson T, Martin R, Kuchroo VK, van Noort JM, Genain CP, Utz PJ, Garren H, Steinman L (2003) Reverse genomics: Protein microarrays guide tolerizing DNA vaccine treatment of autoimmune encephalomyelitis. Nat Biotechnol 21:1033–1039

Ruiz PJ, Garren H, Hirschberg DL, Langer-Gould AM, Levite M, Karpuj MV, Southwood S, Sette A, Conlon P, Steinman L (1999) Microbial epitopes act as altered peptide ligands to prevent EAE. J Exp Med 189:1275–1284

Sakai K, Zamvil SS, Mitchell DJ, Lim M, Rothbard JB, Steinman L (1988) Characterization of a major encephalitogenic T cell epitope in SJL/J mice with synthetic oligopeptides of myelin basic protein. J Neuroimmunol 19:21–32

Smith KJ, Pyrdol J, Gauthier L, Wiley DC, Wucherpfennig KW (1998) Crystal structure of HLA-DR2 (DRA*0101, DRB1*1501) complexed with a peptide from human myelin basic protein. J Exp Med 188(8):1511–1520

Steinman L (2001) Multiple sclerosis: a two stage disease. Nat Immunol 2:762–765

Steinman L (2004) Immune therapy for autoimmune diseases. Science 305:212–216

Steinman L, Conlon P (1997) Viral damage and the breakdown of self-tolerance. Nat Med 3:1085–1087

Tejada-Simon MV, Zang YC, Hong J, Rivera VM, Zhang JZ (2003) Cross-reactivity with myelin basic protein and human herpesvirus-6 in multiple sclerosis. Ann Neurol 53(2):189–197

Ufret-Vincenty R, Quigley L, Tresser N, Pak SH, Gado A, Hausmann S, Wucherpfennig KW, Brocke S (1998) In vivo survival of viral antigen-specific T cells that induce experimental autoimmune encephalomyelitis. J Exp Med 188:1725–1738

Vergelli M, Hemmer B, Utz U, Vogt A, Kalbus M, Tranquill L, Conlon P, Ling N, Steinman L, McFarland H, Martin R (1996) Differential activation of human autoreactive T cell clones by altered peptide ligands derived from myelin basic protein peptide (87–99). Eur J Immunol 26:2624–2634

Warren KG, Catz I, Steinman L (1995) Fine specificity of the antibody response to myelin basic protein in the central nervous system in multiple sclerosis: The minimal B cell epitope and a model of its unique features. Proc Natl Acad Sci USA 92:11061–11065

Warren KG, Catz I, Wucherpfennig KW (1997) Tolerance induction to myelin basic protein by intravenous synthetic peptides containing epitope P85 VVHFFKNIVTP96 in chronic progressive multiple sclerosis. J Neurol Sci 152(1):31–38

Wucherpfennig KW, Catz I, Hausmann S, Strominger JL, Steinman L, Warren KG (1997) Recognition of the immunodominant myelin basic protein peptide by autoantibodies and HLA-DR2 restricted T cell clones from multiple sclerosis patients: Identity of key contact residues in the B-cell and T-cell epitopes. J Clin Invest 100:1114–1122

Wucherpfennig KW, Strominger JL (1995) Molecular mimicry in T cell mediated autoimmunity: viral peptides activate human T cell clones specific for myelin basic protein. Cell 80:695–705

Molecular and Cellular Mechanisms, Pathogenesis, and Treatment of Insulin-Dependent Diabetes Obtained Through Study of a Transgenic Model of Molecular Mimicry

M. B. A. Oldstone (✉)

Division of Virology, Departments of Neuropharmacology and Infectology, The Scripps Research Institute, La Jolla, CA 92037, USA
mbaobo@scripps.edu

1	Introduction	66
2	Experimental Model Designed to Test How Molecular Mimicry Occurs and Produces Virus-Induced Autoimmune IDDM	68
3	Role of the Thymus in Autoimmune Disease	69
4	Molecular Mimicry and Quantitation of Antigen-Specific T Cells Required to Cause IDDM Autoimmune Disease	75
5	Successful Treatment and Prevention of IDDM Autoimmune Disease	79
6	Conclusions	83
References		84

Abstract The portrait of autoimmune diabetes mellitus or type I diabetes can be copied by a transgenic model in which either the nucleoprotein (NP) or glycoprotein (GP) of lymphocytic choriomeningitis virus (LCMV) is expressed in beta cells of the islets of Langerhans. In the absence of further environmental insult, diabetes does not occur. However, when LCMV or a dissimilar virus that shares cross-reactive T cell epitopes with LCMV initiates infection, diabetes ensues. If the self "viral" transgene is expressed only in the beta cells, then diabetes occurs acutely within 8 to 12 days. Specific antiviral (self) CD8 T cells are mandatory for disease, but CD4 T cells are not. In this instance, diabetes can occur in the absence of infection if interferon γ or B7.1 molecules are also expressed in the islets but not when IL-2, IL-4, IL-10, or IL-12 is similarly expressed. In contrast, both CD8 and CD4 antiviral (self) specific T cells are required when the self "viral" transgene is expressed concomitantly in beta cells and in the thymus. In this instance, infection by LCMV or cross-reacting virus is essential to cause diabetes. Further, the time from onset of infection until disease depends, in part, on the host's MHC background and its quantitative influence on negative selection of high-avidity antiviral (self) T cells. Knowledge of the cells, their numbers, and the molecules required to cause diabetes allows the design of successful strategies to treat and prevent the autoimmune disease.

1
Introduction

The autoimmune response is a pathway of the immune response that attacks one's own tissues and causes disease. Most autoimmune diseases are organ (tissue) specific, and they develop when lymphocytes or their products (cytokines, antibodies, perforin, etc.) react with a limited number of antigens in that tissue. The molecular mechanisms leading to autoreactive immune responses resemble those generated when the body acts to expel foreign antigens such as bacteria, parasites, or viruses. However, in autoimmune disease either incomplete clonal deletion or formation of clonal anergy of T and or B cells establishes a population of cells that can, under special circumstances, react with the host's antigens. Self-reactive B cells are deleted in the bone marrow, and self-reactive T cells are eliminated in the thymus, during ontogeny, leaving only those cells that are tolerated by the immune system. Autoimmune disorders are, then, characterized by the breaking of immunologic tolerance or unresponsiveness to self-antigens. Autoimmune diseases affect about 5% of people in developed countries (Bach 2002; Jacobson et al. 1997); however, the incidence of some, such as type 1 diabetes and multiple sclerosis, has significantly increased over the last few years (EURODIAB ACE Study Group 2000; Joy and Johnston 2001; National Diabetes Data Group 1995; Wynn et al. 1990).

Genetic traits and environmental factors as well as the interaction between these elements influence susceptibility to autoimmune diseases (see the chapter on evolution of the concept of molecular mimicry by M.B.A. Oldstone, this volume, for evidence and references). Of all the relevant environmental onslaughts, infection is by far the major initiator or potentiator of autoimmune disorders (Oldstone 1989, 1998; von Herrath et al. 1998, 2002) (Table 1).

Infections trigger autoimmune disease by at least two distinct mechanisms that can function independently or together. One mechanism for understanding how infectious agents cause autoimmunity is molecular mimicry, which is the subject of this volume of *Current Topics in Microbiology and Immunology*. Molecular mimicry in nature is common (Srinivasappa et al. 1986) (see the chapter on evolution of the concept of molecular mimicry by M.B.A. Oldstone, this volume). Experimentally, roughly 5% of monoclonal antibodies generated against a variety of RNA and DNA viruses cross-react with tissue proteins native to test animals. The potential for cross-reactivity of antigens

Infectious Agents Trigger Autoimmune Disease

By activation of autoreactive T cells via:

1. Up-regulation of Th-1 cytokines
   increase of selected molecules: MHC, B7.1, CD28
2. Activation of anti-self (autoimmune) effector T lymphocytes
3. Preferential infection/destruction of CD4 T cell subsets
4. Virus-encoded super-antigens
5. *De novo* release of self epitopes secondary to virus-specific T cell mediated damage: epitope spreading
6. Cross-reactivity with a viral epitope(s): molecular mimicry

Table 1 Mechanisms by which infectious agents trigger autoimmune disease

in host tissues with autoreactive T cells also exists, because a single T cell receptor (TCR) can recognize a broad range of epitopes, including host and viral peptides consisting of sequences that are common to both and those unique to each (Hemmer et al. 2000; Mason 1998). An individual T cell has been calculated to be capable of recognizing more than a thousand distinct peptide epitopes (Mason 1998), although only a few would bind with a sufficient affinity to allow positive selection in the thymus or escape from negative selection with survival in the periphery. Molecular mimicry can also be initiated in other ways. For example, a virus that persists in a selected organ (Oldstone et al. 1984) could serve as a target for the immune response generated later in life after a second virus infection. Experimental evidence for such a scenario was recently suggested by Pinschewer and colleagues (Merkler et al. 2005). Epitope spreading as defined by Sercarz's and Miller's groups provides a means by which cryptic antigen can be uncovered and brought into play after the initial immune attack, thus potentiating related disease by several independent and distinct immune response pathways (McRae et al. 1995; Miller et al. 2001). In contrast and distinct from molecular mimicry, a microorganism may induce autoimmune disease via a bystander activation pathway. Here the mechanism is not antigen specific. Instead, the microbial infection either releases previously sequestered antigens or stimulates cytokines and chemokines, both of which activate antigen-presenting cells and attract lymphoid cells into the target area (Horwitz et al. 1998, 2002). However, the role of bystander cells is still not clear and may vary depending on the experimental system. For example and in contrast to Horwitz's data (Horwitz et al. 1998, 2002), bystander T cell migration to the islets of Langerhans and the CNS without causing tissue injury have also been recorded (Holz et al. 2001; McGavern and Truong 2004; Rhode et al. 2005; von Herrath et al. 1995a).

This review focuses primarily on evidence from the author's laboratory indicating how a virus infection can break immunologic tolerance and, through the mechanism of molecular mimicry, can cause autoimmune insulin-dependent diabetes (IDDM). The work discussed has been carried out over the last 20 years with several gifted colleagues in the Viral-Immunobiology Laboratory, including Peter Southern, Michael Nerenberg, Matthias von Herrath, Jean Edouard Gairin, Andreas Holz, Dirk Homann, Noemi Sevilla, Kurt Edelmann, Urs Christen, Dorian McGavern, Antoinette Tishon, and Hanna Lewicki, as well as with several external colleagues: Marshall Horwitz, Jacques Miller, Nora Sarvetnick, Andrew Luster, Mark Slifka, and Richard Flavell.

2
Experimental Model Designed to Test How Molecular Mimicry Occurs and Produces Virus-Induced Autoimmune IDDM

To better understand the events and molecules involved, we designed a transgenic model and developed the strategy (Oldstone et al. 1991) displayed in Fig. 1. With the rat insulin promoter (RIP), the glycoprotein (GP) or nucleoprotein (NP) of lymphocytic choriomeningitis virus (LCMV) was expressed in the beta (β) cells of the islets of Langerhans of these mice. The GP and NP genes were chosen because they encode the vast majority of dominant and subdominant epitopes recognized by T cells generated during LCMV infection (Ahmed et al. 1984; Riviere et al. 1985, 1986). In contrast, two other LCMV genes are not T cell provocateurs: the polymerase (L), which rarely elicits a T cell response (Lewicki et al. 1992; Riviere et al. 1986), and Z, which up to now has not produced a recognizable response (Homann et al. 2001; Oldstone and Tishon 2004). The general findings of this model are outlined in Fig. 1. In a variation of this model, we expressed the LCMV GP or NP transgene in the thymuses of some transgenic lines as well as in the β cells of their islets (Oldstone et al. 1991; von Herrath et al. 1994b) (Fig. 2). By this means, we were able to evaluate the role of the thymus and the occurrence of autoimmune disease in the presence or absence of negative selection (Fig. 2). Whether or not the RIP-LCMV GP or NP mice had thymic expression of LCMV GP or NP, diabetes did not occur spontaneously (incidence less than 0.01%) unless

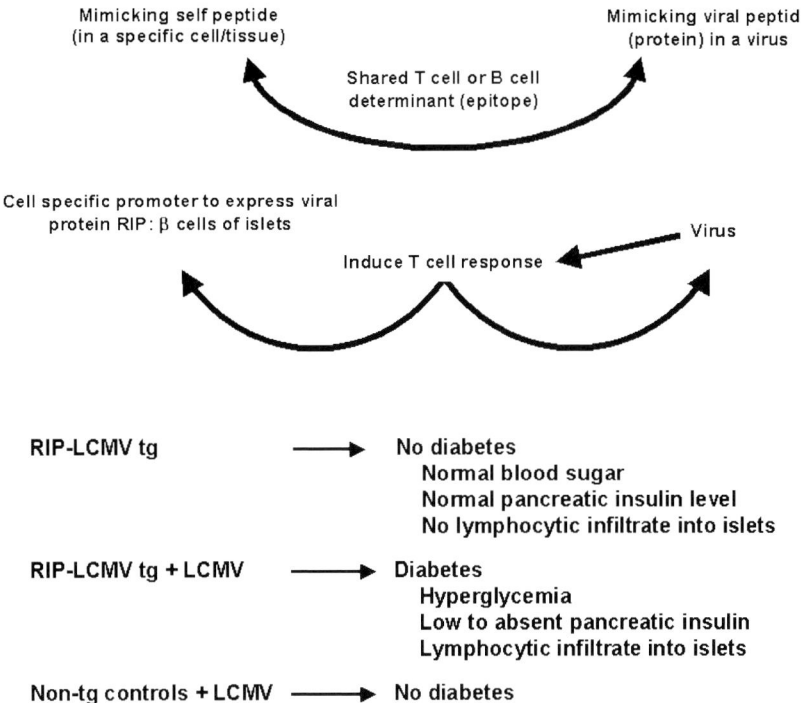

Fig. 1 Cartoon illustrating how a model of IDDM in transgenic mice was caused by molecular mimicry and the phenotype of this disease

tolerance was broken either by viral infection or by other means, as described below, and then the incidence was >90% (Oldstone et al. 1991).

3
Role of the Thymus in Autoimmune Disease

When the transgene was not expressed in the thymus but only in β cells of the islets of Langerhans, potentially autoreactive T cells of high affinity passed through the thymus by positive selection and migrated to the periphery (von Herrath et al. 1995b) (Fig. 3). Under these circumstances, tolerance could be spontaneously broken by interferon (IFN)-γ or B7.1 expressed in the β cells (Lee et al. 1995; von Herrath et al. 1995b), resulting in diabetes. However, the expression of neither interleukin (IL)-2 nor IL-12 was able to break tolerance (Holz et al. 2001; von Herrath et al. 1995a). On challenge with LCMV, tolerance was broken, and IDDM followed within 7–12 days in RIP-LCMV mice.

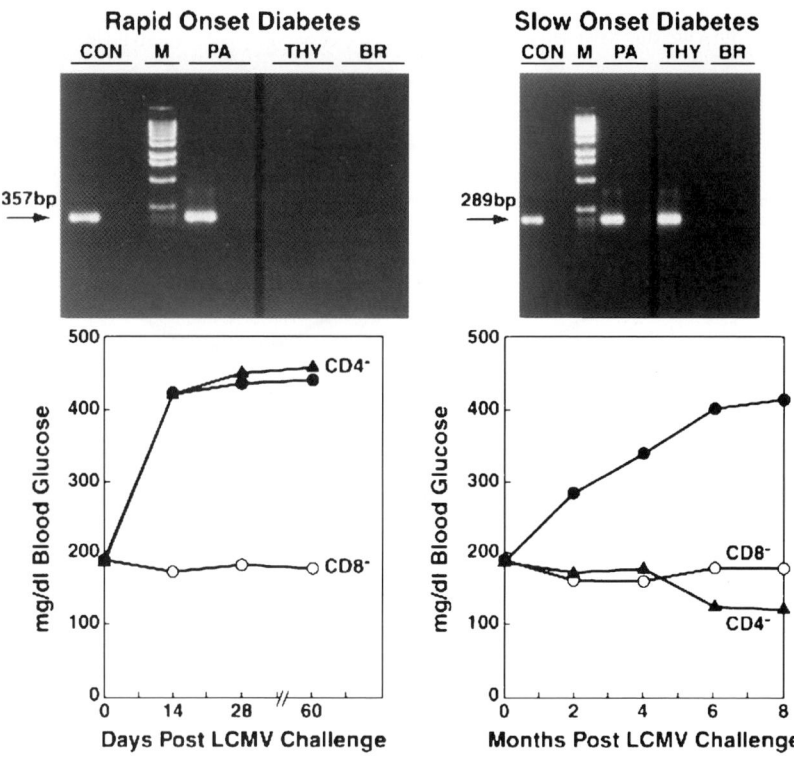

Fig. 2 Role of the thymus in the kinetics of IDDM establishment and in CD8+ T cell-dependent but CD4+ T cell-independent injury. When the viral transgene is expressed only in pancreatic β cells, disease occurs rapidly within 7 to 12 days after viral infection and requires only CD8 T cells as observed in RIP-LCMV mice lacking CD4 or CD8 T cells (knockout background) or after depletion of either CD4 or CD8 T cell populations with monoclonal antibodies specific to each. In contrast, when the transgene is expressed in the thymus as well as the β cells, the onset of disease is slower, i.e., IDDM occurs in months instead of days. Further, CD4 and CD8 antigen-specific T cells are both required (see von Herrath et al. 1994b)

This IDDM did not require CD4 T cell participation; only CD8 T cells were needed (Laufer et al. 1993; von Herrath et al. 1994b) (Fig. 2). The mechanism involved is displayed in Fig. 3. Figure 4 lists the molecules we found that could break tolerance in the absence of viral infection or effectively enhance the autoimmune disease in association with viral infection. These studies were performed on double transgenic mice that expressed the molecule(s) shown in Fig. 4 along with the viral transgene solely in the β cells of the islets of Langerhans (Holz et al. 2001; Lee et al. 1994, 1995; Mueller et al. 1995, 1996;

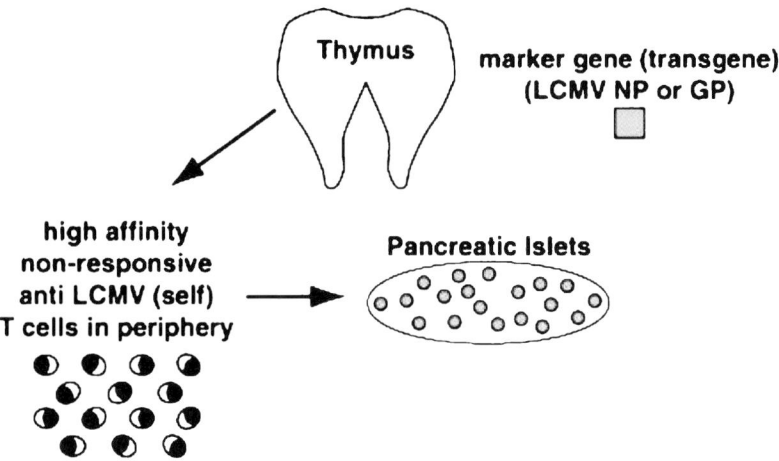

Component 1: Tropism and Preparation of Target Organ

1. **Cytokine expression by β cells**: sufficient for activation of anti "self" T cells and causing IDDM

2. **LCMV virus infection of islets**: required (a) to prepare local milieu of cytokine/chemokine expression, MHC + costimulatory molecules + integrin upregulation; (b) activate and expand anti "self" T cells; (c) migration of antigen-presenting cells to pancreatic lymph nodes and islets

Fig. 3 Activation of positively selected high-affinity antiviral (self) autoimmune cells in the periphery causes acute-onset IDDM. In this scenario, the transgene (viral, self) determinant is in the β cells of the islets of Langerhans but not in the thymus

von Herrath and Oldstone 1997; von Herrath et al. 1995a, 1995b). A similar transgenic model of acute autoimmune diabetes was simultaneously developed and reported by Ohashi and colleagues (Ohashi et al. 1991). However, both models recapitulate the less common form of this autoimmune disease, e.g., rapid-onset IDDM. Instead, autoimmune diseases commonly take several months or years to develop after the initial stimuli. Our model in which the cross-reactive epitope lies both in the thymus and in the target organ (Figs. 2, 5) best mirrors autoimmune diseases like IDDM. T cells are essential in causing IDDM; neither B lymphocytes nor antibodies are needed (Holz et al. 2000).

Summary of Cytokine Studies in RIP LCMV Transgenics

Breakage of peripheral tolerance (ignorance)		Enhancement of autoimmune disease	
+	IFN-γ	+	IFN-γ
	B-7.1		B-7.1
			IL-2
NIL	IL-2		IL-12
	IL-12		
	IL-4	NIL	IL-4
	IL-10		IL-10

Fig. 4 Summary of data from double-transgenic mice. The molecules displayed are expressed under control of the RIP promoter and then crossed to RIP LCMV transgenic mice and are associated with the spontaneous development of IDDM with or without virus infection. In these mice, infection enhances the kinetics and severity of IDDM

The thymus played two other essential roles. The first role is the relationship between MHC haplotype and thymic control over negative selection. For these studies, the LCMV NP gene was expressed in the thymus with the Thy1.2 promoter (von Herrath et al. 1994a). On primary challenge with LCMV, H-2^d Balb and H-2^b C57Bl/6 mice, not expressing LCMV NP in their thymi, mounted a cytotoxic T lymphocyte (CTL) response to an immunodominant domain of the NP at aa 118–127 and aa 396–405, respectively. In the transgenic mice with LCMV NP expressed in their thymi, this high-affinity CD8 CTL response was deleted but a low-affinity NP CTL response was made. Dilutions of H-2^b or H-2^d NP peptide indicated that 3 to 4 logs less of the H-2^b NP peptide were required to sensitize syngeneic target cells for CTL-specific lysis than that needed by the H-2^d NP peptide. In contrast, equivalent amounts of both peptides were required to sensitize target cells taken from normal, non-Thy1.2 NP transgenic mice. When the LCMV NP transgene was expressed in both the thymus and islet β cells, the H-2^b mice developed IDDM sooner (1–2 months)

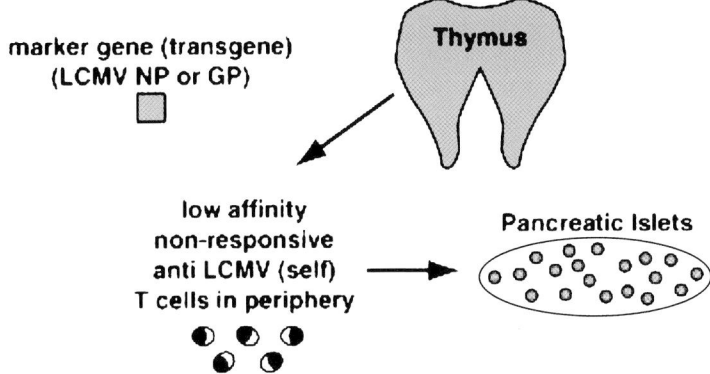

Component 1: Tropism and Preparation of Target Organ

1. <u>Cytokine expression by β cells</u>: <u>unlable</u> to activate anti "self" T cells or cause IDDM unless anti "self" T cell pool is expanded with LCMV infection

2. <u>LCMV virus infection of islets</u>: required (a) to prepare local milieu of cytokine/chemokine expression, MHC + costimulatory molecules + integrin upregulation; (b) activate and expand anti "self" T cells; (c) migration of antigen-presenting cells to pancreatic lymph nodes and islets

Component 2: Potentiation of Ongoing Autoimmune Disease

1. <u>Infection by non-related DNA or RNA</u> virus that share X-reactive T cell epitopes with "self" (LCMV) further activate and expand anti "self" T cells

Fig. 5 Cartoon of steps involved in causing autoimmune disease with low-affinity antiviral (self) T cells in the periphery. In this scenario the transgene (virus, self determinant) is expressed both in the β cells of the islets of Langerhans and in the thymus

than $H-2^d$ mice (3–4 months) or $H-2^k$ mice (6 months); the latter also required less peptide than $H-2^b$ mice for sensitization. Thus MHC control over thymic selection helps to dictate the numbers and affinities of antigen-specific T cells in the periphery. This, in turn, is associated with the kinetics (1–2 vs. 3–4 vs. 6 months) and severity ($H-2^b > H-2^d > H-2^k$) of ensuing disease.

The second essential role of the thymus in this context is its impact on the avidity of T cell responders. We had noted a choice of subdominant CD8 T cells for preferential escape from negative selection, resulting in alteration of the antiviral T cell hierarchy (Slifka et al. 2003; von Herrath et al. 1994a) (Fig. 6). As an example, in H-2^d mice infected with LCMV Armstrong (ARM), the immunodominant viral epitope is NP aa 118–126, whereas the subdominant epitopes are GP 283–292 and NP 313–321. When we created transgenic mice that expressed LCMV ARM NP in the thymus, CD8 T cells specific for the subdominant epitope NP 313 were essentially unaffected by thymic and/or positive selection. In contrast, the T cell response against the dominant epitope NP 118 was significantly compromised in terms of both functional avidity and structural avidity. The functional response was quantitated by stimulation with subsaturating amounts of peptides or activation by various peptide analogs. The avidity of the dominant T cell populations could be determined by peptide-tetramer binding assays (Slifka et al. 2003). In terms of negative selection events that occurred in vivo, three important points were uncovered. First, $CD8^+$ T cells specific for subdominant epitopes escaped virtually unscathed from negative selection in the thymus and peripheral organs. Second, the most promiscuous $CD8^+$ T cells specific for an immunodominant self-

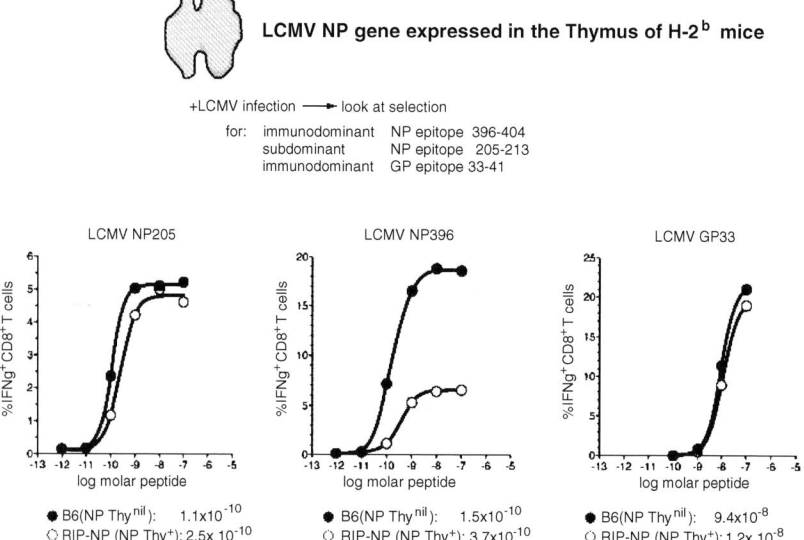

Fig. 6 Negative selection of CD8 T cells in the thymus alters the hierarchy of the antiviral (self) autoaggressive cells (see Slifka et al. 2003; von Herrath et al. 1994a)

epitope were deleted during negative selection. Third, CD8⁺ T cells specific for dominant epitopes were deleted as a function of their structural avidity, but this deletion caused no major changes in expression levels of TCR or in the family of $V\beta$ genes used. Thus the process of negative selection narrows the structural diversity of the peripheral T cell pool, but without necessarily leading to unacceptable defects within the TCR repertoire.

4
Molecular Mimicry and Quantitation of Antigen-Specific T Cells Required to Cause IDDM Autoimmune Disease

Molecular mimicry is not necessary for but can play a role in the activation of high-affinity antiviral (self) autoimmune T cells in the periphery (Fig. 3). However, molecular mimicry is essential for the expansion and activation of low-affinity antiviral (self) autoimmune T cells in the periphery (Fig. 5). In addition, the initiating virus must be tropic for the target organ attacked by the immune cells. This local infection prepares the tissue for an eventual autoimmune assault (von Herrath and Holz 1997). These events are portrayed in Fig. 5. This assault is specific, as we showed by using RIP-LCMV NP H-2^b (Balb) transgenic mice in which the LCMV ARM NP is expressed in the thymus and β cells and low-affinity anti-LCMV NP (self) autoimmune T cells are in the periphery. As Fig. 7 illustrates, only infection with LCMV strains ARM or E350 can cause IDDM (defined as a blood glucose level above 300 mg/dl) in a CD8 sufficient mouse (Fig. 7). Diverse RNA and DNA viruses like Coxsackie, vaccinia, herpes simplex (not shown), or Pichinde cannot. Similarly, LCMV strains Pasteur and Traub, which share over 95% homology of NP with ARM and E350, cannot elevate blood glucose levels or cause CTL migration into the islets to cause IDDM. As quantitated by limiting dilution analysis, at least one antigen-specific CD8⁺ cell per approximately 1,000 total CD8 T cells is required to cause IDDM. The Pasteur strain of LCMV fails to make sufficient CTL to cause IDDM because it has three amino acid mutations in the single immunodominant NP epitope 118–127, with L substituting for P at aa 119, K for Q at aa 120, and T for A at aa 121. The Traub strain has a NP 118–127 sequence homologous with that of ARM and E350 but substitutes an A for a T at position 131. Transfection studies show that this mutation in the COO⁻ flanking region significantly alters intracellular processing of the Traub NP (Sevilla et al. 2000). Yet Traub, Pasteur, E350 and ARM strains of LCMV all cross-react with each other at the T cell level at the NP aa 118–128 CD8 epitope. Thus the inability to generate sufficient effector CTL for cross-reacting viruses that fail to cause IDDM can be mapped to point mutations in the CTL epitope

To expand sufficient antigen-specific "antiself" T cells in the periphery to cause disease need to activate adoptive immune response by molecular mimic.

Quantifiable number of antigen-specific T cells required to cause disease.

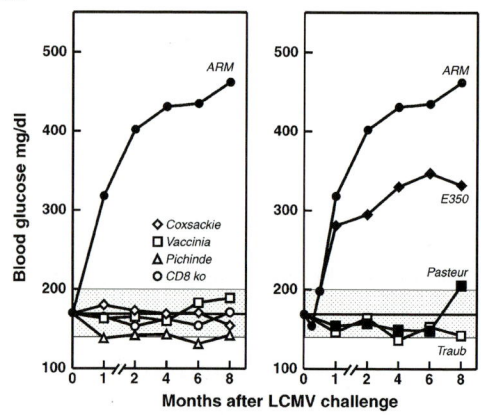

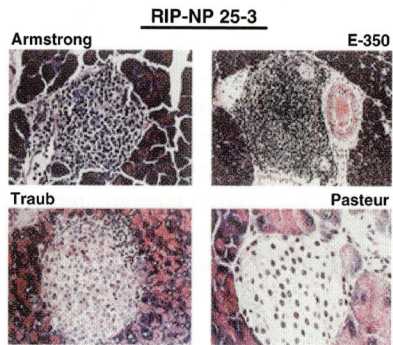

Virus Inoculum	pcf CTL (ARM-NP) / RIP 25-3 ARM-NP	Incidence IDDM
Arm	810	++++
E350	1078	+++
Traub	8000	nil
Pasteur	15,800	nil
Coxsackie	0	nil
Vaccinia	0	nil
Pichinde	0	nil

Fig. 7 Both specificity and a quantifiable number of antigen-specific T cells are required to cause the autoimmune disease

per se or its COO⁻ flanking region. *These important data indicate that neither the standard epidemiological markers nor molecular analysis with nucleic acid probes currently in use reliably distinguish among viruses that do or do not cause IDDM and that the same likely holds true for other autoimmune diseases.*

Recently, Dorian McGavern established a quantitative assay for evaluating the migration and deposition of antigen-specific CD8 T cells required to cause disease (McGavern et al. 2002). For this technique, one crosses transgenic mice that express green fluorescent protein (GFP) under a beta actin promoter with transgenic mice having immunodominant H-2D^b-restricted LCMV CD8 TCR. The double-positive cells are isolated and adoptively transferred into syngeneic RIP LCMV mice. On LCMV challenge, the TCR (GFP staining) cells rapidly expand by several magnitudes and move to the target area. This assay allows direct counting of migrating and target-resident antigen-specific CD8 cells (or CD4 T cells when GFP-expressing mice are crossed to TCR CD4 cells) in the organ afflicted with autoimmune disease. According to this assay, approximately four million antigen-specific CD8 T cells must occupy the islets to cause IDDM (Christen et al. 2004b).

Definitive evidence for molecular mimicry causing IDDM in the RIP-LCMV model, as cartooned in Fig. 5, was recently observed when H-2^b transgenic mice inoculated with Pichinde virus failed to develop the expected IDDM yet did so when inoculated with LCMV ARM (Figs. 7, 8A). The cause of this IDDM had absolute immunologic specificity, i.e., the source was CTL against the immunodominant H-2^b D^b-restricted LCMV ARM NP epitope aa 396–404. This conclusion was confirmed when a variant LCMV ARM with L substituted for F at aa 403 failed to cause IDDM (Fig. 8A) and also failed to elicit a virus-specific CD8 CTL response (Lewicki et al. 1995a, 1995b). As anticipated, removal of the effector CD8 T cells genetically or with anti-CD8 T cell antibody aborted the ability of LCMV ARM to cause IDDM. However, in a two-step protocol with LCMV given first to activate low-affinity anti-LCMV NP (self) CD8 T cells, followed 3 to 4 weeks later by exposure to Pichinde virus, the incidence of IDDM over that caused by LCMV inoculation alone was accelerated and enhanced (Christen, Edelmann et al. 2004b) (Fig. 8B). It was subsequently shown that the K^b-restricted Pichinde virus epitope NP aa 205–212 YTVKFPNM dramatically enhanced a subdominant LCMV NP epitope NP aa 205–212 YTVKYPNL (Fig. 8C) as initially shown by Ray Welsh. When these studies were repeated on K^b knockout mice, neither the NP

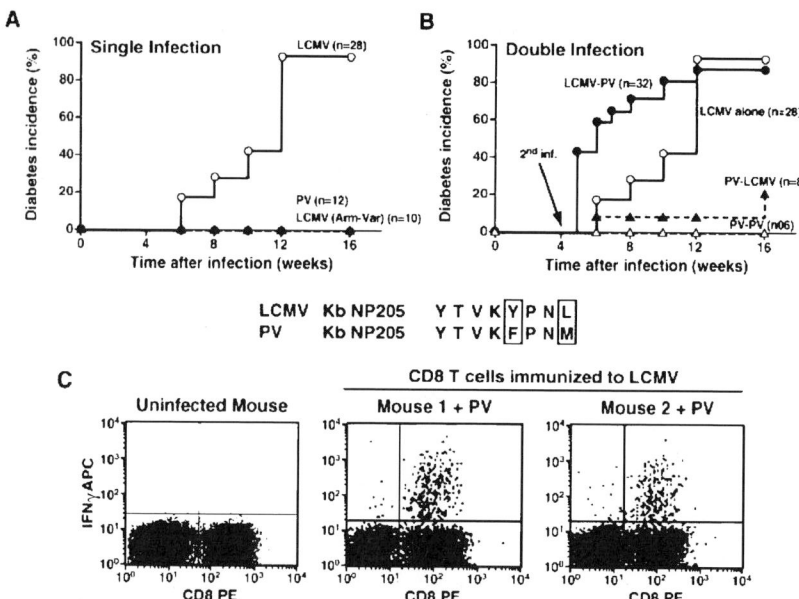

Fig. 8A–C Molecular mimicry accelerates autoimmune IDDM by expanding cross-reactive CD8 T cells that interact with the subdominant domain of NP aa 205–212 of Pichinde virus and with LCMV ARM (see Christen et al. 2004b for details). A Inoculation of RIP LCMV-NP mice that contain the NP transgene in both the thymus and pancreatic β cells with 1×10^5 PFU of LCMV ARM causes IDDM in 90% of mice (28 per group) by 12 weeks. The immunodominant epitope is NP aa 396–404. Inoculation of 1×10^5 variant LCMV ARM that contains a single aa substitution in this epitope is unable to generate LCMV-specific NP CTL and cannot cause IDDM. However, this variant LCMV generates CTL to GP epitopes (see references in Lewicki et al. 1995a, 1995b). Inoculation of 1×10^5 Pichinde virus (PV) fails to cause IDDM after a 20-week observation period. **B** When PV is given 4 weeks after primary LCMV ARM CTL in RIP LCMV-NP transgenic mice, 50% of mice develop IDDM by 5 weeks of age as compared to 50% of mice given LCMV ARM requiring 12 weeks. In contrast, administering PV followed by LCMV or another inoculation of PV results in less than 7% of mice developing IDDM over a 16-week observation period. **C** Expansion of NP 205 CTL by molecular mimicry. Numbers of NP 205–212 CTL are enhanced in LCMV-primed recipients of PV inoculation 4 weeks later (data for two mice shown; mouse 1 LCMV primed + PV, mouse 2 LCMV primed + PV). This response is K^b- not D^b restricted, and Pichinde virus-induced IDDM does not occur in K^b knockout mice (see Christen et al. 2004b). The expansion and migration of these additional K^b-restricted NP aa 205–212 CD8 antigen-specific T cells to the islets of Langerhans can be detected by using a tetramer technique (see Christen et al. 2004b). As a result, the number of specific autoaggressive CD8 T cells increases to the level required to kill sufficient β cells to cause IDDM

205–212 CTL response nor the IDDM occurred after Pichinde virus infection (Christen et al. 2004b). Further, with the use of tetramer technology to mark antigen-specific CD8 T cells in the islet tissue in K^bD^b sufficient mice given the double infection of LCMV ARM followed by Pichinde virus, it was noted that K^b-specific CD8 T cells were absent in K^b knockout mice that failed to develop IDDM but were present in K^b-sufficient mice that became diabetic.

5
Successful Treatment and Prevention of IDDM Autoimmune Disease

Understanding and quantitating the events underlying IDDM in the RIP-LCMV model allowed us to design therapeutic approaches to prevent or halt this virus-induced autoimmune disease. Table 2 lists the successful procedures and the mechanistic basis of their functions. Briefly, when the cytokine profile in the islet of Langerhans milieu was changed from a Th1 to a Th2 phenotype (IFN-γ to IL-4, IL-10, TGF-β), IDDM was blocked (Homann et al. 1999; Lee et al. 1994, 1996; Mueller et al. 1995, 1996; von Herrath et al. 1996). One interesting way this occurred was through the oral administration of porcine insulin (Fig. 9, left upper panel) (Homann et al. 1999; von Herrath et al. 1996). This therapy had no demonstrable effect on the precursor frequency of effector $CD8^+$ CTL. However, when a single or double amino acid change was made in the β chain of the insulin molecule that ordinarily protected against IDDM, the protective effect was lost, and some preparations even enhanced

Treatment and Prevention

1. **Change islet milieu from Th1 to Th2 cytokine profile abort IDDM**
   i. prevent IFN-γ expression (ko)
   ii. enhance IL-4 expression (RIP tg)
   iii. oral insulin therapy: prevents IDDM by decreasing expression IFN-γ and enhancing expression IL-4 bearing lymphocytes

2. **Specifically block IDDM producing T cells**
   i. peptide therapy

3. **Specifically block disease associated MHC allele expression**
   i. E3 transcription complex of adenovirus (RIP tg)

Table 2. Successful therapies to treat and prevent IDDM

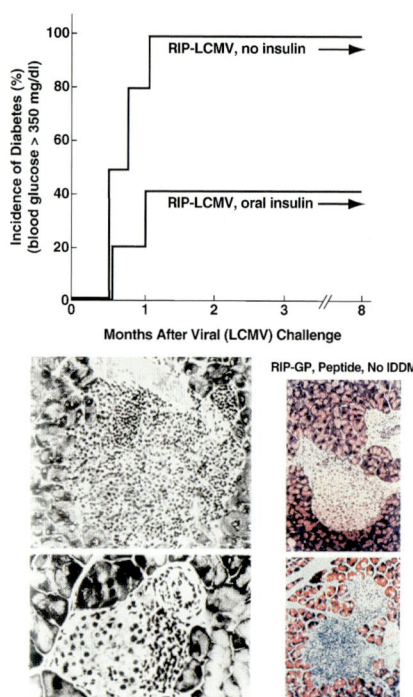

Treatment with Db-Binding SMIENLEYM Blocking Peptide
Prevents LCMV Induced IDDM in RIP-LCMV Transgenic Mice

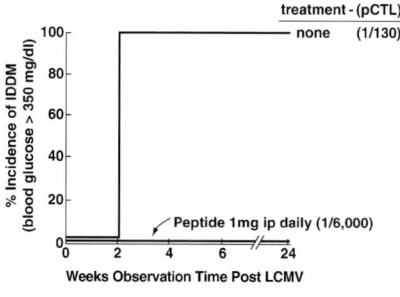

		nM	CTL
CTL antagonist	S M I E N L E Y M	5 ± 2	NIL
GP aa 33-41	K A V Y N F A T C	21 ± 4	+++
GP aa 276-286	S G V E N P G G Y C L	13 ± 3	+++
NP aa 396-404	F Q P Q N G Q F I	6 ± 1	+++

Fig. 9 Oral insulin or inoculation of a designer peptide successfully blocks the occurrence of IDDM. *Left upper panel:* Oral injection of insulin prevents IDDM by altering the islet milieu with a decrease of T lymphocytes expressing IFN-γ replaced by T lymphocytes expressing IL-4 (see Homann et al. 1999; von Herrath et al. 1996). *Lower panel*: Creation of a designed peptide capable of blocking natural D^b epitopes for CD8 T cells (see Oldstone et al. 1999). *nM*, 50% inhibition, with a value of <50 nM being a good binder. The engineered peptide is able to block CTL-mediated killing by the three immunodominant CTL epitopes displayed. *Right upper panel:* The designer peptide, when administered to RIP-LCMV NP $H-2^b$ mice, aborts the expected IDDM after inoculation of such mice with LCMV. Here the numbers of effector CTLs is significantly reduced from 1 antigen-specific CD8 T cell per 130 total CD8 T cells to 1 antigen-specific T cell to 6,000 total CD8 T cells, thereby abrogating the diabetic onset

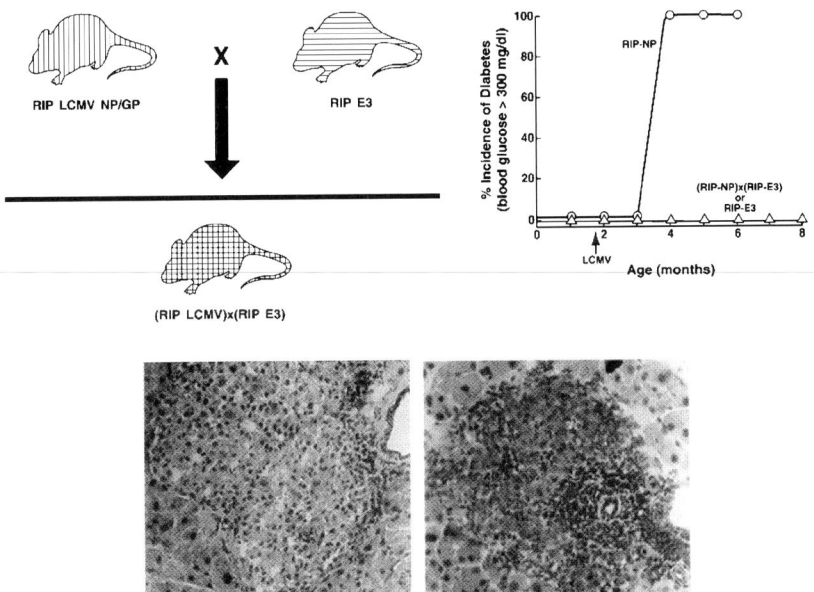

Fig. 10 Expression of the E3 transcriptional complex of adenovirus in β cells of the islets of Langerhans aborts IDDM in RIP-LCMV mice. *Left upper panel:* Generation of double-transgenic mice. *Right upper panel*: The expression of E3 in β cells prevents IDDM (see von Herrath et al. 1997). Subsequent experiments implicate the GP-19 transcriptional unit as likely responsible for downregulating the relevant MHC molecule. *Lower panel*: Lack of migratory lymphocytes (*left*) in a RIP LCMV×RIP E3 transgenic mouse treated with LCMV. In the *lower right panel*, lymphocytes are clearly visible in a similarly treated single transgenic RIP LCMV mouse

the IDDM. In the latter instances, transgenic mice got IDDM within 1 week after LCMV challenge. This outcome documents how little we know about what controls immunity vs. tolerance with respect to oral therapy. A second approach was to design a peptide that bound at high affinity to the MHC allele involved in IDDM (Fig. 9, lower panel) (Oldstone et al. 1999). After administration of this reagent, IDDM did not occur; although CD4$^+$ and CD8$^+$ T cells were not found in the islets (Fig. 9, upper right panel). What this peptide therapy accomplished was to reduce the numbers of antigen-specific T cells so that too few remained to cause IDDM. A third approach was to abort expression of the MHC class I molecule by expressing the E3 transcription complex of adenovirus in β cells with the RIP promoter (Fig. 10) (von Herrath et al. 1997). The focal reduction of MHC class I expression in the islets was associated with a normal precursor frequency of CD8$^+$ CTL. Effector T cells did not accumulate in the islets, so IDDM did not develop. Preliminary studies

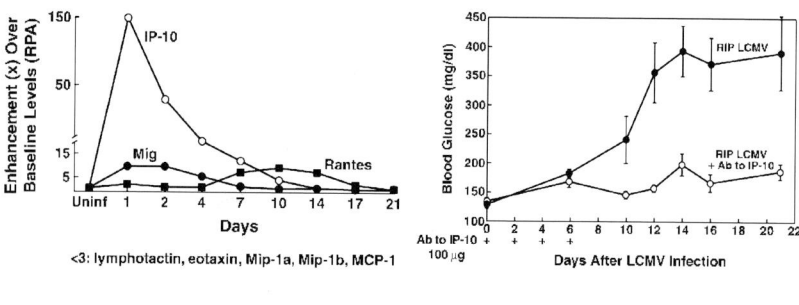

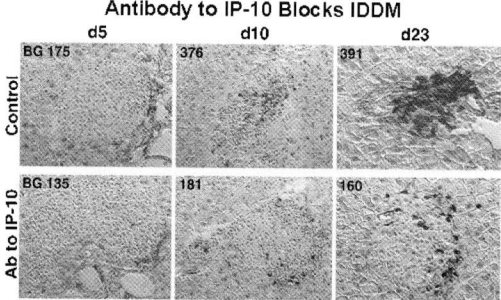

Fig. 11 Neutralization of the chemokine IP-10 produced in the islets after virus infection aborts the expansion and migration of lymphocytes into the islets and prevents IDDM (see Christen et al. 2004a). The induction of IP-10 in the islets in vivo within 24 h after LCMV infection is shown in the *upper left panel*. Note the lower levels of other chemokines in the islets at this time. Treatment with antibody to IP-10 diminishes the migration of antigen-specific T cells into the islets (*lower panel*) and aborts the expected occurrence of IDDM (*right upper panel*)

with Marshall Horwitz using RIP E3×RIP-LCMV transgenic mice in which various transcription factors of E3 gene were knocked out suggested that deletion of GP-19, which decreases MHC molecules but leaves intact FAS and TNF-α, aborts the protective effect of the E3 gene. When, instead, the transcripts for TNF and FAS were deleted but GP-19 remained intact, the E3 gene kept its protective effect.

A fourth therapeutic approach was to discourage the expansion and migration of antigen-specific T cells to the islet target tissue. This was accomplished by using antibody to IP-10 (Christen et al. 2004a). Within the first 24 h of an initial infection with LCMV, we noted that IP-10 levels were enhanced nearly 200-fold over baseline values in the islets (Fig. 11, left panel). Our subsequent treatment with neutralizing antibodies to IP-10 (Christen et al. 2004a) prevented the expansion and migration of antigen-specific T cells to the target tissue and to the islets of Langerhans (Fig. 11, lower panel), thereby aborting the otherwise inevitable IDDM (Fig. 11, right panel).

6
Conclusions

Infectious agents, particularly viruses, are implicated in autoimmunity on the basis of three findings. The first is that autoimmune responses made de novo or those already present are enhanced by infection with a wide variety of human DNA and RNA viruses. This point is strengthened by the second finding that, in several experimental animal models, both acute and persistent virus infections can induce, accelerate, or enhance autoimmune responses and cause autoimmune disease. Third, with an investigative approach that focuses on one potential mechanism whereby microbes cause autoimmunity, i.e., molecular mimicry, a number of etiologic agents have been defined as potential causes of autoimmune disease.

Analysis of molecular mimicry in an animal model of IDDM reveals several important concepts that challenge how current epidemiological surveys are employed to seek the causative agents of human autoimmune diseases. First, the initiating event (viral infection) absolutely must begin the autoimmune process, but, in most instances, this instigator is gone from the host by the time that autoimmune disease becomes manifested (a hit-and-run phenomenon). One or multiple infections that follow are or may be by themselves not sufficient to directly cause autoimmune disease but, by eliciting a cross-reactive immune response, can enhance the number of activated antiself T cells to the levels necessary for disease. Thus epidemiological studies carried out not at the earliest stage, but instead when disease is overt, are unlikely to identify the initiating agent. Finally, a few point mutations in the T cell epitope or in the flanking sequences allow one to detect viruses that cross-react immunologically and are definable in Northern or Western blots, but the cross-reaction, per se, is inefficient in generating the numbers of antigen-specific T cells required to cause disease. Thus serological profiling and gene probes as currently used to seek the etiologic agents of diabetes and other autoimmune disease will likely miss the agent(s) of interest that cause the disease.

Finally, and importantly, because a quantifiable number of antigen-specific autoreactive cells are an absolute requirement to cause autoimmune injury and disease, the design and use of strategies that limit and reduce that number, even when not depleting all the autoaggressive cells, should be effective in treating and preventing autoimmune attacks, as well as enhancing the survival of islet grafts.

Acknowledgements This is Publication Number 17030-NP from the Department of Neuropharmacology, The Scripps Research Institute, La Jolla, CA. This work was supported in part by USPHS Grants DK-058541, AI-009484, and AI-045927.

References

Ahmed R, Byrne JA, Oldstone MBA (1984) Virus specificity of cytotoxic T lymphocytes generated during acute lymphocytic choriomeningitis virus infection: Role of the H-2 region in determining cross-reactivity for different lymphocytic choriomeningitis virus strains. J Virol 51:34–41

Bach JF (2002) The effect of infections on susceptibility to autoimmune and allergic diseases. N Engl J Med 347:911–920

Christen U, Benke D, Wolfe T, Rodrigo E, Rhode A, Hughes AC, Oldstone MBA, von Herrath MG (2004a) Cure of prediabetic mice by viral infection involves lymphocyte recruitment along an IP-10 gradient. J Clin Invest 113:74–84

*Christen U, *Edelmann KH, McGavern DB, Wolfe T, Coon B, Teague MK, Miller SD, Oldstone MBA, von Herrath MG (2004b) A viral epitope that mimics a self antigen can accelerate but not initiate autoimmune diabetes. J Clin Invest 114:1290–1298
*Contributed equally to this work

EURODIAB ACE Study Group (2000) Variation and trends in incidence of childhood diabetes in Europe. Lancet 355:873–876

Hemmer B, Jacobsen M, Sommer N (2000) Degeneracy in T-cell antigen recognition: implications for the pathogenesis of autoimmune diseases. J Neuroimmunol 107:148–153

Holz A, Brett K, Oldstone MBA (2001) Constitutive β cell expression of IL-12 does not perturb self-tolerance but intensifies established autoimmune diabetes. J Clin Invest 108:1749–1758

Holz A, Dyrberg T, Hagopian W, Homann D, von Herrath M, Oldstone MBA (2000) Neither B lymphocytes nor antibodies directed against self antigens of the islets of Langerhans are required for development of virus-induced autoimmune diabetes. J Immunol 165:5945–5953

Homann D, Dyrberg T, Petersen J, Oldstone MBA, von Herrath MG (1999) Insulin in oral immune "tolerance": a one-amino acid change in the B chain makes the difference. J Immunol 163:1833–1838

Homann D, Teyton L, Oldstone MBA (2001) Differential regulation of antiviral T-cell immunity results in stable $CD8^+$ but declining $CD4^+$ T-cell memory. Nat Med 7:913–919

Horwitz MS, Bradley LM, Harbertson J et al (1998) Diabetes induced by Coxsackie virus: initiation by bystander damage and not molecular mimicry. Nat Med 4:781–785

Horwitz MS, Ilic A, Fine C, Rodriguez E, Sarvetnick N (2002) Presented antigen from damaged pancreatic beta cells activates autoreactive T cells in virus-mediated autoimmune diabetes. J Clin Invest 109:79–87

Jacobson DL, Gange SJ, Rose NR, Graham NM (1997) Epidemiology and estimated population burden of selected autoimmune diseases in the United States. Clin Immunol Immunopathol 84:223–243

Joy JE, Johnston Jr RB (eds) (2001) Committee on multiple sclerosis: Current status and strategies for the future. Board on Neuroscience and Behavioral Health. The National Academies Press, Washington, DC

Laufer TM, von Herrath MG, Grusby MJ, Oldstone MBA, Glimcher LH (1993) Autoimmune diabetes can be induced in transgenic major histocompatibility complex class II-deficient mice. J Exp Med 178:589–596

Lee M-S, Sawyer S, Arnush M, Krahl T, von Herrath M, Oldstone MBA, Sarvetnick N (1996) Transforming growth factor-beta fails to inhibit allograft rejection or virus-induced autoimmune diabetes in transgenic mice. Transplantation 61:1112–1115

Lee M-S, von Herrath M, Reiser H, Oldstone MBA, Sarvetnick N (1995) Sensitization to self (virus) antigen by in situ expression of murine interferon-γ. J Clin Invest 95:486–492

Lee M-S, Wogensen L, Shizuru J, Oldstone MBA, Sarvetnick N (1994) Pancreatic islet production of murine interleukin-10 does not inhibit immune-mediated tissue destruction. J Clin Invest 93:1332–1338

Lewicki H, McKee T, Tishon A, Salvato M, Whitton JL, Oldstone MBA (1992) Novel LCMV specific $H-2^k$ restricted CTL clones recognize internal viral gene products and cause CNS disease. J Neuroimmunol 41:15–20

Lewicki H, Tishon A, Borrow P, Evans C, Gairin JE, Hahn KM, Jewell DA, Wilson IA, Oldstone MBA (1995a) CTL escape viral variants. I. Generation and molecular characterization. Virology 210:29–40

Lewicki HA, von Herrath MG, Evans CF, Whitton JL, Oldstone MBA (1995b) CTL escape viral variants. II. Biologic activity in vivo. Virology 211:443–450

Mason D (1998) A very high level of crossreactivity is an essential feature of the T-cell receptor. Immunol Today 19:395–404

McGavern D, Christen U, Oldstone MBA (2002) Molecular anatomy of antigen-specific CD8+ T cell engagement and synapse formation in vivo. Nat Immunol 3:918–925

McGavern D, Truong P (2004) Rebuilding an immune-mediated central nervous system disease: Weighing the pathogenicity of antigen-specific versus bystander T cells. J Immunol 173:4779–4790

McRae BL, Vanderlugt CL, Dal Canto MC, Miller SD (1995) Functional evidence for epitope spreading in the relapsing pathology of experimental autoimmune encephalomyelitis. J Exp Med 182:75–85

Merkler D, Horvath E, Bruck W, Zinkernagel RM, de la Torre JC, Pinschewer DD (2005) "Dual viral hit" mimics organ-specific autoimmunity. Personal communication. Submitted.

Miller SD, Olson JK, Croxford JL (2001) Multiple pathways to induction of virus-induced autoimmune demyelination: lessons from Theiler's virus infection. J Autoimmun 16:219–227

Mueller R, Krahl T, Sarvetnick N (1996) Pancreatic expression of interleukin-4 abrogates insulitis and autoimmune diabetes in nonobese diabetic (NOD) mice. J Exp Med 184:1093–1099

Mueller R, von Herrath M, Oldstone MBA, Sarvetnick N (1995) Expression of IL-4 in β cells of the islets of Langerhans aborts insulin dependent diabetes mellitus in a transgenic model. Unpublished observations.

National Diabetes Data Group (1995) Diabetes in America, 2nd Edition. National Institutes of Health, National Institute of Diabetes and Digestive and Kidney Diseases. NIH Publication No. 95-1468, Bethesda, MD

Ohashi P, Oehen S, Buerki K et al (1991) Ablation of tolerance and induction of diabetes by virus infection in viral antigen transgenic mice. Cell 65:305–317

Oldstone MBA (1989) Virus induced autoimmunity: Molecular mimicry as a route to autoimmune disease. J Autoimmun 2:187–194

Oldstone MBA (1998) Molecular mimicry and immune-mediated diseases. FASEB J 12:1255–1265

Oldstone MBA, Nerenberg M, Southern P, Price J, Lewicki H (1991) Virus infection triggers insulin-dependent diabetes mellitus in a transgenic model: Role of anti-self (virus) immune response. Cell 65:319–331

Oldstone MBA, Southern P, Rodriguez M, Lampert P (1984) Virus persists in beta cells of islets of Langerhans and is associated with chemical manifestations of diabetes. Science 224:1440–1443

Oldstone MBA, Tishon A (2004) Unpublished results.

Oldstone MBA, von Herrath M, Lewicki H, Hudrisier D, Whitton JL, Gairin JE (1999) Use of a high-affinity peptide that aborts MHC-restricted cytotoxic T lymphocyte activity against multiple viruses in vitro and virus-induced immunopathologic disease in vivo. Virology 256:246–257

Rhode A, Pauza M, Rodrigo E, Oldstone MBA, von Herrath MG, Christen U (2005) Islet-specific expression of CXCL10 causes spontaneous islet infiltration and accelerates diabetes development. J Exp Med, submitted.

Riviere Y, Ahmed R, Southern PJ, Buchmeier MJ, Dutko FJ, Oldstone MBA (1985) The S RNA segment of lymphocytic choriomeningitis virus codes for the nucleoprotein and glycoproteins 1 and 2. J Virol 53:966–968

Riviere Y, Southern PJ, Ahmed R, Oldstone MBA (1986) Biology of cloned cytotoxic T lymphocytes specific for lymphocytic choriomeningitis virus. V. Recognition is restricted to gene products encoded by the viral S RNA segment. J Immunol 136:304–307

Sevilla N, Homann D, von Herrath M, Rodriguez F, Harkins S, Whitton JL, Oldstone MBA (2000) Virus-induced diabetes in a transgenic model: Role of cross-reacting viruses and quantitation of effector T cells needed to cause disease. J Virol 74:3284–3292

Slifka MK, Blattman JN, Sourdive DJ, Liu F, Huffman DL, Wolfe T, Hughes A, Oldstone MBA, Ahmed R, von Herrath MG (2003) Preferential escape of subdominant CD8+ T cells during negative selection results in an altered antiviral T cell hierarchy. J Immunol 170:1231–1239

Srinivasappa J, Saegusa J, Prabhakar BS, Gentry MK, Buchmeier MJ, Wiktor TJ, Koprowski H, Oldstone MBA, Notkins AL (1986) Molecular mimicry: frequency of reactivity of monoclonal antiviral antibodies with normal tissues. J Virol 57:397–401

von Herrath M, Dockter J, Oldstone MBA (1994b) How virus induces a rapid or slow onset insulin-dependent diabetes mellitus in a transgenic model. Immunity 1:231–242

von Herrath M, Holz A (1997) Pathological changes in the islet milieu precede infiltration of islets and destruction of beta-cells by autoreactive lymphocytes in a transgenic model of virus-induced IDDM. J Autoimmun 10:231–238

von Herrath MG, Allison J, Miller JFAP, Oldstone MBA (1995a) Focal expression of interleukin-2 does not break unresponsiveness to "self" (viral) antigen expressed in β cells but enhances development of autoimmune disease (diabetes) after initiation of an anti-self immune response. J Clin Invest 95:477–485

von Herrath MG, Dockter J, Nerenberg M, Gairin JE, Oldstone MBA (1994a) Thymic selection and adaptability of cytotoxic T lymphocyte responses in transgenic mice expressing a viral protein in the thymus. J Exp Med 180:1901–1910

von Herrath MG, Dyrberg T, Oldstone MBA (1996) Oral insulin treatment suppresses virus-induced antigen-specific destruction of β cells and prevents autoimmune diabetes in transgenic mice. J Clin Invest 98:1324–1331

von Herrath MG, Efrat S, Oldstone MBA, Horwitz MS (1997) Expression of adenoviral E3 transgenes in beta cells prevents autoimmune diabetes. Proc Natl Acad Sci USA 94:9808–9813

von Herrath MG, Guerder S, Lewicki H, Flavell RA, Oldstone MBA (1995b) Coexpression of B7.1 and viral ("self") transgenes in pancreatic β cells can break peripheral ignorance and lead to spontaneous autoimmune diabetes. Immunity 3:727–738

von Herrath MG, Holz A, Homann D, Oldstone MBA (1998) Role of viruses in type I diabetes. Semin Immunol 10:87–100

von Herrath MG, Homann D, Oldstone MBA (2002) The role of viruses. In: Gill RG, Harmon JT, Maclaren NK (eds) Immunologically mediated endocrine diseases. Lippincott Williams & Wilkins, Philadelphia, pp 639–665

von Herrath MG, Oldstone MBA (1997) Interferon-γ is essential for destruction of β cells and development of insulin-dependent diabetes mellitus. J Exp Med 185:531–539

Wynn DR, Rodriguez M, O'Fallon WM, Kurland LT (1990) A reappraisal of the epidemiology of multiple sclerosis in Olmsted County, Minnesota. Neurology 40:780–786.

Trypanosoma cruzi-Induced Molecular Mimicry and Chagas' Disease

N. Gironès · H. Cuervo · M. Fresno (✉)

Centro de Biología Molecular, CSIC-UAM, Universidad Autónoma de Madrid, Cantoblanco, 28049 Madrid, Spain
Mfresno@cbm.uam.es

1	**Chagas' Disease**	90
1.1	General Aspects and Life Cycle	90
1.2	Clinical Findings	91
1.3	Immune Response	93
2	**Chronic Chagasic Cardiopathy**	94
2.1	Pathological Findings	94
2.2	Mechanisms of Pathogenesis	94
2.3	Immunological Findings	95
3	**Autoimmunity and Infection**	97
4	**Autoimmunity in *T. cruzi* Infection**	98
5	**Molecular Mimicry**	99
5.1	Mimetic B Cell Epitopes	99
5.1.1	Myosin	99
5.1.2	Ribosomal Proteins	103
5.1.3	Cha	104
5.2	Autoreactive T Cells	106
6	**Bystander Activation**	108
7	**Parasite Persistence**	109
8	**Coexistence of Parasite Persistence and Autoimmunity**	112
9	**Final Remarks**	113
	References	114

Abstract Chagas' disease, caused by *Trypanosoma cruzi*, has been considered a paradigm of infection-induced autoimmune disease. Thus, the scarcity of parasites in the chronic phase of the disease contrasts with the severe cardiac pathology observed in approximately 30% of chronic patients and suggested a role for autoimmunity as the origin of the pathology. Antigen-specific and antigen-non-specific mechanisms have been described by which *T. cruzi* infection might activate T and B cells, leading to autoimmunity. Among the first mechanisms, molecular mimicry has been claimed as the most important mechanism leading to autoimmunity and pathology in the chronic phase of this disease. In this regard, various *T. cruzi* antigens, such as B13, cruzipain and Cha, cross-react with host antigens at the B or T cell level and their role in pathogenesis has been widely studied. Immunization with those antigens and/or passive transfer of autoreactive T lymphocytes in mice lead to clinical disturbances similar to those found in Chagas' disease patients. On the other hand, the parasite is becoming increasingly detected in chronically infected hosts and may also be the cause of pathology either directly or through parasite-specific mediated inflammatory responses. Thus, the issue of autoimmunity versus parasite persistence as the cause of Chagas' disease pathology is hotly debated among many researchers in the field. We critically review here the evidence in favor of and against autoimmunity through molecular mimicry as responsible for Chagas' disease pathology from clinical, pathological and immunological perspectives.

Abbreviations

Ag(s)	Antigen(s)
IFN	Interferon
CTL	Cytotoxic T lymphocyte
IL	Interleukin
TNF	Tumor necrosis factor
mAb	Monoclonal antibody
iNOS	Inducible nitric oxide synthase
DTH	Delayed-type hypersensitivity
TCR	T cell receptor
ECM	Extracellular matrix
MHC	Major histocompatibility complex
Mhc	Myosin heavy chain
CMhc	Cardiac myosin heavy chain
SMhc	Skeletal myosin heavy chain
APC(s)	Antigen-presenting cell(s)
ICAM	Intercellular adhesion molecule
CCC	Chronic chagasic cardiompathy
VCAM	Vascular cell adhesion molecule

1
Chagas' Disease

1.1
General Aspects and Life Cycle

Chagas' disease (Chagas 1909) is a debilitating multisystemic disorder which affects several million people (approximately 18 million individuals are infected with *Trypanosoma. cruzi*, with 120 million at risk) in Central and South America (Moncayo 1999; Prata 2001; Tanowitz et al. 1992) and is considered a paradigm of infection-mediated autoimmune disease. It is caused by the flagellated protozoan parasite *Trypanosoma cruzi*, with a complex life cycle involving several stages in both vertebrates and insect vectors. *T. cruzi* has three main different morphologies: epimastigote, which replicates in the blood-sucking triatomine insect vector; trypomastigote, which infects the vertebrate host's cells; and amastigote, which replicates intracellularly in the host's cells (Burleigh and Andrews 1998; Tanowitz et al. 1992).

Transmission of *T. cruzi* to humans occurs when feces released by the bug while it takes a blood meal, containing infective metacyclic trypomastigote forms of the parasite penetrate, into the bloodstream, where the metacyclic forms infect a wide variety of host phagocytic and non-phagocytic cells. Once inside the cells, the metacyclic forms escape from endocytic vacuoles to the cytoplasm, where they transform into amastigotes, which multiply intracellularly (see Fig. 1 for details).

Individuals residing in rural areas of Latin America are at highest risk of infection, because the bugs live in these dwellings and feed on the inhabitants at night. The World Health Organisation has conducted several programs for the elimination of the insect vector, with great results on the incidence of new infections (Moncayo 1999). On the other hand, transfusion-acquired Chagas' disease is becoming a significant health problem in countries other than Central and South America, especially those receiving high numbers of immigrants from that region (Kirchhoff 1989; Wendel 1998).

1.2
Clinical Findings

Two phases, acute and chronic, can be differentiated in Chagas' disease (Kirchhoff 1993; Prata 2001; Tanowitz et al. 1992). In the acute phase, encompassing a few weeks after infection, a local inflammatory lesion appears at the site of infection, where the metacyclic trypomastigotes infect and undergo their first rounds of multiplication. After parasite dissemination through the body, circulating blood trypomastigotes are easily observed in blood (parasitemia) and a small number of patients develop symptoms of cardiac insufficiency, reflecting an underlying severe myocarditis, leading, in some instances, to heart failure responsible for the few deaths in acute Chagas' disease (Dias et al. 1956; Prata 1994). Meningoencephalitis may also occur, especially in some immunosuppressed patients (Hoff et al. 1978). However, the acute phase mostly remains undiagnosed without severe clinical symptoms. In contrast, the severe pathology and the most common manifestations of this disease develop

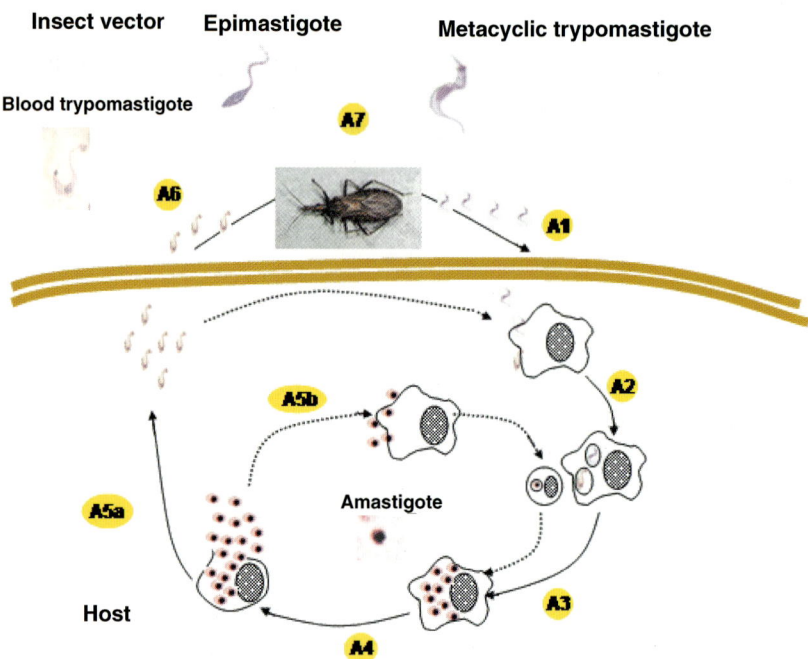

Fig. 1 Infective cycle of *Trypanosoma cruzi*. Transmission of *T. cruzi* to humans occurs when feces released by the bug while it takes a blood meal and containing infective metacyclic trypomastigote forms of the parasite (*A1*) penetrate into the bloodstream, where they infect a wide variety of host phagocytic and non-phagocytic cells (*A2*). Once inside the cells, the metacyclic forms escape from endocytic vacuoles to the cytoplasm, where they transform into amastigotes, which multiply intracellularly (*A3*). At some point, the amastigotes break off from the cell (*A4*) and differentiate into non-replicative flagellated blood trypomastigotes which in turn can penetrate and infect adjacent susceptible cells or spread to infect cells and tissues at distant locations of the body (*A5a*). Amastigotes can also directly infect phagocytic cells (*A5b*). Muscle cells, including those of the heart, are amongst the most heavily infected. Circulating trypomastigotes may be taken up by a new triatomine bug during a blood meal (*A6*). Inside the vector's intestine, ingested blood trypomastigotes differentiate into replicative epimastigotes, which, as they move to the mid and lower gut, transform into non-replicative but infective metacyclic trypomastigotes

many years (10 to 30) after the initial infection with *T. cruzi* in the so-called chronic phase, although only in 30%–40% of the infected people (Kirchhoff 1993; Prata 2001; Tanowitz et al. 1992). During the chronic phase, circulating parasites cannot be observed by inspection of blood but progressive tissue damage occurs involving the esophagus, colon and heart (Prata 2001; Tanowitz et al. 1992). Treatment with benznidazol or nifurtimox is effective during the acute phase of infection, but no treatment exists for the chronic phase (Prata 2001; Tanowitz et al. 1992). To date, an effective immunotherapy or vaccine is still lacking.

1.3
Immune Response

The immune response against this parasite is complex and far from being clearly established. Both humoral and cellular immune responses are involved in controlling *T. cruzi*, which is not surprising because of the complexity of the parasite's life cycle. Thus, although B cell-deficient mice succumb to infection (Kumar and Tarleton 1998), the protective immune response seems to depend on $CD8^+$ T cells that produce interferon (IFN)-γ. $CD8^+$ T cells can control the infection through cytotoxic T lymphocyte (CTL)-induced perforin/granzyme-mediated killing of infected cells and/or FAS-mediated apoptosis (Kumar and Tarleton 1998). However, there are reports indicating that $CD8^+$ T cells cannot completely control infection because they become unresponsive (Martin and Tarleton 2004). Cytokines play a key role in regulating both the induction and type of immune response as well as parasite replication in infected hosts (Fresno et al. 1997). Macrophages, which can be infected by *T. cruzi*, also play a crucial role in the elimination of this parasite. Activation of monocytes by cytokines released by Th1 cells seems to be a key process in controlling infection in vitro as well as in vivo. Thus, Interleukin (IL)-12 produced by macrophages in response to infection mediates resistance to *T. cruzi* (Aliberti et al. 1996). Tumor necrosis factor (TNF)-α and IFN have been identified as the most important cytokines involved in the killing of intracellular *T. cruzi* through an NO-mediated-L-arginine dependent killing mechanism (Gazzinelli et al. 1992; Muñoz-Fernandez et al. 1992). This was corroborated in vivo, because anti-IFN-γ monoclonal antibody (mAb) administration results in a drastic increase in parasitemia and mortality (Silva et al. 1992; Torrico et al. 1991). Moreover, mice deficient for IFN-γ receptor and inducible nitric oxide synthase (iNOS) had an increased susceptibility to infection and parasitemia (Holscher et al. 1998; Goni et al. 2002), although the role of NO has been recently disputed because some iNOS-deficient mice do not seem to be more susceptible to infection (Laucella et al. 2004). TNF-R1-FcIgG$_3$ transgenic mice are also more susceptible to *T. cruzi* infection, clearly indicating a protective role for TNF-α (Castanos-Velez et al. 1998).

2
Chronic Chagasic Cardiopathy

2.1
Pathological Findings

The most important pathology of Chagas' disease develops 10–30 years after primary infection and affects several internal organs, mainly, heart, esophagus and colon, as well as the peripheral nervous system. The heart is the organ most commonly involved; cardiopathy frequently develops, congestive heart failure being a common cause of death in these patients. Megaesophagus and/or megacolon may also develop in chronic chagasic patients, which in the most severe form can cause life-threatening malnutrition and intractable constipation. Chronic chagasic cardiopathy (CCC) is thus the most devastating manifestation of Chagas' disease. However, despite affecting about a third of the infected people the pathogenesis of CCC is still poorly understood.

CCC may be considered a progressive disease, in which myocardial inflammation and fibrosis plays a pivotal role (Carrasco Guerra et al. 1987; Higuchi et al. 1987; Pereira Barretto et al. 1986). Higher percentages of severe myocarditis, fibrosis and myocardial hypertrophy are found in CCC patients with heart failure compared to patients in the indeterminate phase and with cardiac arrhythmia. Examination of the hearts of CCC patients who have died of heart failure shows biventricular enlargement with occasional apical aneurysms. In addition, individuals with CCC often develop mural thrombi, which may cause cerebrovascular accidents. Histological examination of the heart reveals diffuse interstitial fibrosis, lymphoid infiltration and damaged myocytes, all occurring in the apparent absence of parasites. Fibrosis and chronic inflammation are also detected in the conduction system of the heart, which may account for the high incidence of arrhythmias.

2.2
Mechanisms of Pathogenesis

Despite intensive research, the etiology of Chagas' heart disease, both in humans and in experimental animal models of the disease, is not clearly understood. Although the acute and chronic phases of the disease share some similar pathological findings, it is still unclear whether similar pathogenic mechanisms operate. In this regard, infiltration by $CD4^+$ T cells seems to take place in the acute phase of the disease, whereas $CD8^+$ T cells predominate in the chronic phase (Henriques-Pons et al. 2002). Moreover, it is plausible that the pathology of the acute phase may affect the final outcome of the chronic phase.

To date, many pathogenic mechanisms have been described to explain how cardiac pathology develops. They can be mediated directly by the parasite or caused by an inflammatory/immune/autoimmune mechanism or a combination of these. These mechanisms are summarized below:

- *Primary neuronal damage* resulting in denervation of the parasympathetic autonomous system in the heart. This was one of the first pathogenic mechanisms described during the acute phase (Koberle 1961, 1970). However, subsequent studies only show slight neuronal damage in the heart, suggesting that neuronal lesions are an epiphenomenon, secondary to inflammation and fibrosis (Davila et al. 1991, 2002; Rossi 1996).
- *T. cruzi-induced damage to cardiomyocytes,* due to the cytopathic effect caused by intracellular infection with amastigotes or by the release of secreted *T. cruzi* product(s), which can be toxic for host cells and tissues (Koberle and Nador 1955). This is an obvious mechanism, but may have only some relevance in the acute phase and in heavily parasitized or immunosuppressed patients.
- *Parasite-induced microvascular changes* may lead to cardiac hypoperfusion and finally to myocyte degeneration and chronic inflammation (Factor et al. 1985; Morris et al. 1990; Petkova et al. 2001).
- *Persisting T. cruzi antigens* may act as trigger for specific $CD4^+$ or $CD8^+$ T-cell mediated responses of either the delayed-hypersensitivity (DTH) type or cytotoxic $CD8^+$ cells that lead to damage to infected cells or to bystander cells in the host tissues (Ben Younes-Chennoufi et al. 1988; Tarleton 2001; Tarleton and Zhang 1999). This mechanism may take place in both the acute and the chronic phase.
- *Autoimmunity* may occur by a variety of mechanisms (listed in Table 1). Those could be due to *T. cruzi* antigen (Ag)-specific mechanisms (molecular mimicry) or non-parasite Ag-specific effector mechanisms and are discussed in detail below.

An important point which is often ignored in this debated field is that none of the mechanisms listed above is mutually exclusive. Moreover, it seems unlikely that heart damage can be attributed to only one of these mechanisms.

2.3
Immunological Findings

In CCC, 50% macrophages, 40% T cells with a predominance of $CD8^+$ over $CD4^+$ T cells and 10% B cells comprise the inflammatory infiltrate

Table 1 Mechanisms for activation of T and B cells in autoimmune diseases

a. Microbial antigen specific:
- Molecular mimicry between parasite and host antigens triggers autoimmunity
- Bystander activation (TCR dependent)

b. Microbial antigen non-specific:
- Release of autoantigen(s) during an infection
- Bystander activation (TCR independent)
- Cryptic epitopes
- Superantigens

(Cunha-Neto et al. 2004). T cell receptor (TCR) Vβ transcripts are heterogeneous in heart biopsies from CCC patients (Cunha-Neto et al. 1994) which is a characteristic of other well-defined autoimmune diseases. The number of $CD4^+$ T cells increased in parallel to the number of $CD8^+$ T cells in acute-phase but not in chronic-phase patients with heart failure, suggesting an immunological imbalance.

Cytokines and chemokines produced in response to the parasite may upregulate vascular cell adhesion molecule (VCAM)-1 and intercellular adhesion molecule (ICAM)-1, increased on endothelial cells of patients, which recruit $VLA-4^+LFA-1^+CD8^+$ T lymphocytes (dos Santos et al. 2001). In this regard, a role for cell adhesion molecules and integrin receptors, extracellular matrix (ECM) components, matrix metalloproteinases and chemokines has been proposed in the differential recruitment and migration in infected hosts of *T. cruzi*-elicited $CD8^+$ and inflammatory cells into the heart and other susceptible host tissues (Marino et al. 2003a, 2003b). It is worth noting that ECM components may absorb parasite Ags and cytokines which could contribute to the establishment and perpetuation of inflammation. Moreover, we have found that *T. cruzi* requires β1 integrins to gain access to the cell (Fernandez et al. 1993). The inflammatory response, which is probably recurrent, undergoing periods of more accentuated exacerbation, is most likely responsible for progressive neuronal damage, microcirculation alterations, heart matrix deformations and consequent organ failure.

CCC patients have increased expression of major histocompatibility complex (MHC) molecules. Thus, class I MHC are upregulated in the sarcolemma of myocytes in the myocardium (Higuchi Mde et al. 2003) and there is also evidence for an over-expression of class II MHC in endothelial cells (Benvenuti et al. 2000; Laucella et al. 1999; Reis et al. 1993). This may favor the presentation of cryptic epitopes to infiltrating T cells.

3
Autoimmunity and Infection

Two main classes of mechanisms have been described by which infectious agents might activate T and B cells, leading to autoimmunity: Ag-specific and Ag-non-specific (Table 1). The Ag-specific mechanisms mostly state that sequence similarity between infectious agents and self-proteins (molecular mimicry or epitope mimicry) is responsible for the triggering of the autoimmune response (Oldstone 1989; Penninger and Bachmaier 2000; Rose 2001; Rose and Mackay 2000; Wucherpfennig 2001). Autoreactive B and/or T cells, in response to foreign Ags originated by molecular mimicry, can arise from a T/B cell cooperation mechanism, but experimental direct evidence is still scarce (Oldstone 1989; Rose and Mackay 2000). However, there are as yet no absolute formal proofs demonstrating that molecular mimicry is the initiating event of human autoimmune disease and responsible for the pathology, as noted recently (Benoist and Mathis 2001; Fourneau et al. 2004). Probably, Chagas' disease is close to that paradigm. There is some consensus that in order to prove the involvement of epitope mimicry in a disease of suspected autoimmune etiology five criteria must be demonstrated experimentally (Benoist and Mathis 2001; Kierszenbaum 1986) (see Table 2).

The microbial Ag-non-specific theory has several variations. The common characteristic is that no particular microbial determinant is implicated, although the infection may be the initial event which triggers the autoimmune reaction. For example, infection might cause host cell destruction, which results in the release of large quantities of normally sequestered Ags. Those cryptic epitopes found in intracellular proteins are not normally presented in the context of Class I MHC and are therefore not normally encountered by host lymphocytes. These Ags could then be captured by dendritic cells that migrate to T cell areas of the lymphoid organs, where they trigger naïve T cells, or presented at the invasion site, leading to activation of autoreactive cells (but

Table 2 Criteria required for demonstration of the involvement of molecular mimicry in a disease of suspected autoimmune etiology

---

1. Association of the disease with a particular microorganism
2. Identification of the culprit microorganism epitope that elicits the cross-reactive response
3. T or B cell populations against that epitope should be expanded in the infection
4. Elimination of the cross-reactive epitope from the microorganism should result in non-pathogenic infection
5. Autoreactive T cells should be able to transfer the disease

not against the infecting microorganism). In addition, cryptic epitopes may initiate and maintain autoimmunity through various non-mutually exclusive mechanisms (Lanzavecchia 1995). Those cryptic epitopes can be presented by non-professional Ag-presenting cells (APCs, such as B cells) and induce T cell activation. Autoreactive B cells initiate autoimmunity in the absence of T cells specific for the self-Ag. Alternatively, autoreactive B cells may take up a foreign Ag that cross-reacts with a self-Ag at the B cell level but contains different T cell epitopes. Finally, activated B cells, which efficiently take up and present self-Ag, may prime autoreactive T cells. All these mechanisms may result in a self-sustained autoimmune response.

Microbial infection may result in bystander activation, which may take place in the setting of a proinflammatory milieu. Thus microbial infection induces the release of proinflammatory cytokines such as TNF and chemokines which could be able to activate autoreactive T cells by lowering the threshold of activation (Kim and Teh 2001; Vakkila et al. 2001). These T cells may then proliferate in response to self-Ags presented on host APCs. Inflammation could also alter lymphocyte migration patterns and activate APCs, rendering them more effective as APCs by enhancing Ag uptake and processing, cell surface expression of major MHC molecules, or costimulatory molecules. Finally, infection might provoke polyclonal lymphocyte activation via either a mitogen or a super-Ag effect (Stauffer et al. 2001).

4
Autoimmunity in *T. cruzi* Infection

The finding of a T cell-rich inflammatory mononuclear cell infiltrate and the scarcity of parasites in heart lesions questioned the direct participation of *T. cruzi* in CCC and suggested the possible involvement of autoimmunity, although this remains a hotly debated issue (Engman and Leon 2002; Kierszenbaum 1986, 1999; Levin 1996; Soares et al. 2001; Tarleton 2001, 2003). Several early studies on Chagas' disease already emphasized the scarcity of parasites in histological sections in the chronic phase of the disease (Andrade and Andrade 1955; Mazza 1949). Since then, much research in the field has focused on the possibility that autoimmune responses set off by molecular mimicry and/or bystander activation contribute to tissue damage. Those mechanisms were initially reported many years ago (Acosta and Santos-Buch 1985; Cossio et al. 1984, 1974a, 1974b; McCormick and Rowland 1989; Santos-Buch and Teixeira 1974; Takle and Hudson 1989; Wood et al. 1982) and they were supported by a large body of circumstantial evidence thereafter and have been extensively and sequentially reviewed (Eisen and Kahn 1991; Engman and Leon 2002; Kierszenbaum 1986, 1999; Leon and Engman 2001; Soares et al. 2001). Although the presence of "anti-self" immune responses in *T. cruzi* infections has been unquestionably demonstrated, the case of the mediation of cross-reactive antibodies or T cells in pathology is still far from settled. Taking into account the variety of the mechanisms of induction of autoimmunity shown in Table 1 the relevant question is, Which mechanisms can be applied to *T. cruzi* infection?

On the other hand, mounting evidence is challenging this view. Thus, with the use of more sensitive techniques, parasite Ags or parasite DNA has been detected during the chronic phase, attributing all the damage either to an inflammatory response against the parasite or to the parasite replication itself (reviewed in Tarleton 2001, 2003; Tarleton and Zhang 1999). It should be emphasized that to date there is no unequivocal demonstration that either autoimmunity or parasite-specific immunity is pathogenic.

5
Molecular Mimicry

The detection of circulating anti-*T. cruzi* antibodies that cross-react with host heart and neural Ags is a common finding in chagasic humans and animal models of infection (reviewed in Engman and Leon 2002; Kierszenbaum 1999, 2003) but, with few exceptions, none of the autoantibodies seems to be the leading cause of autoimmune pathogenesis. In *T. cruzi* infection many examples of molecular mimicry at the level of T cells or antibodies have been described (recently reviewed in Cunha-Neto et al. 2004). However, few of these have been extensively studied and/or defined at the molecular level (see Table 3). We will focus our review only on those examples.

5.1
Mimetic B Cell Epitopes

5.1.1
Myosin

Probably the most studied cross-reactive autoantigen in Chagas' disease is myosin. Several *T. cruzi* Ags have been shown to cross-react with myosin (cardiac or skeletal muscle) and have been implicated in pathogenesis through molecular mimicry. Cunha-Neto and collaborators have described cardiac myosin heavy chain (CMhc) as a major Ag of heart-specific autoimmunity and suggested the possible relevance of myosin recognition in human CCC (Cunha-Neto et al. 1995; Kalil and Cunha-Neto 1996). Antibodies to CMhc

Table 3 Molecular mimicry described during *T. cruzi* infection. Defined and partially defined cross-reactive epitopes

	Cross-reactive antigens	Cross-reactive epitopes	Molecular definition	Reference
Host *T. cruzi*	Cardiac myosin heavy chain (CMhc) B13	AAALDK ::: :: AAAGDK	Ab T cells	Abel et al. 1997
Host *T. cruzi*	23-kDa ribosomal protein Ribosomal protein (R13)	EESD(D/E)DMGFGLFD ::: : :::::::: EEED D DMGFGLFD	Ab	Levitus et al. 1991
Host *T. cruzi*	β1 Adrenergic receptor Ribosomal protein P0	AESDE ::: : AESEE	Ab	Ferrari et al. 1995
Host *T. cruzi*	β1 Adrenergic receptor[a] M2 muscarinic receptor[a] Ribosomal protein (R13)	--ED-D-GF-LFD[a] --EDDDMGF-LFD[a] EEEDDDMGFGLFD	Ab	Mahler et al. 2004
Host *T. cruzi*	47-kDa neuron protein FL-160	TPQRKTTEDRPQ	Ab	Van Voorhis et al. 1991
Host *T. cruzi*	Cha antigen Shed acute-phase antigen (SAPA)	SLVTCPAQGSLQSSPSMEI : . :: : :..:: . STPSTPADSSAHSTPSTPV	T cells	Girones et al. 2001b
Host *T. cruzi*	Cha antigen TENU2845/36 kDa	MRQLDTNVER . : : : : : : . LRQLDF-VEE	Ab	Girones et al. 2001a, 2001b

[a] Residues of the R13 epitope that when interacting with purified antibodies trigger stimulation of the denoted receptor.

were found in symptomatic as well as asymptomatic patients. Affinity-purified anti-CMhc antibodies specifically recognized two polypeptides of 140,000 and 116,000 Da in *T. cruzi* trypomastigotes. At the molecular level, cross-reactivity was shown to exist between the amino acid sequence AAALDK of CMhc and the AAAGDK sequence from a recombinant *T. cruzi* peptide named B13 (Table 3). All sera from patients with CCC disease, but only 14% of sera from asymptomatic chagasic patients, recognized B13 (Gruber and Zingales 1993). These results have been often disputed, although no contradictory results have been published (see Kierszenbaum 2003). However, there were some discrepancies between the 100% reactivity of the sera from chronic patients with overt heart disease with CMhc and only 61% reactivity in those with *T. cruzi*, a finding difficult to reconcile with molecular mimicry.

Cruzipain, a well-defined and highly abundant *T. cruzi* Ag, is involved in CCC pathogenesis by various direct and indirect mechanisms. The latter are also related to cross-reactivity with myosin, although not with CMhc but with skeletal muscle myosin heavy chain (SMhc). Thus purified anti-cruzipain antibodies raised in cruzipain-immunized mice cross-react with SMhc (Giordanengo et al. 2000a, 2000b) and, more importantly were associated with heart conduction disturbances in those animals. Moreover, ultrastructural findings revealed severe alterations of cardiomyocytes and IgG deposit on heart tissue of immunized mice. Giordanengo et al. investigated whether antibodies induced by cruzipain transferred from immunized mothers to their offspring could alter the heart function in the pups. All IgG isotypes against cruzipain derived from transplacental crossing were detected in pups' sera. Electrocardiographic studies performed in the offspring born to immunized mothers revealed conduction abnormalities (Giordanengo et al. 2000b). These results provide strong evidence for a pathogenic role of the humoral autoimmune response induced by a purified *T. cruzi* Ag in the development of experimental Chagas' disease. More recently, Sterin-Borda et al. have reported that immunization with cruzipain also induces autoantibodies against muscarinic acetylcholine receptors which can be implicated in pathology (Sterin-Borda et al. 2003). However, in both cases described above the molecular identification of cross-reactive epitopes of cruzipain and host proteins is still lacking.

On the other hand, *T. cruzi*- infected A/J mice (a strain of mice highly susceptible to *T. cruzi* infection) generated anti-myosin IgG, both in the acute phase and the chronic phase of infection (Leon et al. 2001). Moreover, heart lesions resembling those seen in *T. cruzi*-infected mice can be induced by immunization with purified myosin. However, not all mouse strains are equally susceptible to myocytolysis after *T. cruzi* infection (Leon and Engman 2001). Interestingly, in C57BL/6 mice, the levels of anti-myosin IgG found after *T. cruzi* infection were small or undetectable and no myocarditis was observed in the acute phase (Leon et al. 2001). Moreover, the C57BL/6 mouse strain has been claimed not to develop cardiac autoimmunity after immunization with myosin (Neu et al. 1987). These results suggest that generation of anti-myosin antibodies by *T. cruzi* infection or myosin immunization depends on the genetic background of the host and that there is a clear relationship between anti-myosin IgG and heart damage. However, from these results it is unclear whether anti-myosin IgG is the cause or the effect of heart damage. Accordingly, we have seen that C57BL/6 mice infected with *T. cruzi* did not develop clinically relevant myocarditis in the acute phase. However, at 120 days after infection, C57BL/6 mice developed a milder myocarditis compared to mice deficient for iNOS gene with the same genetic background (Girones et al. 2004). Because C57BL/6 developed lower parasitemias than iNOS knockout mice in the acute phase, this may be taken as an indication that the presence or absence of myocarditis may depend on the initial level of control of parasite replication rather than on the genetic background of the host.

In contrast to the above, other reports suggested that anti-myosin antibodies are not involved in the pathogenesis. For example, immunization with myosin in immunosuppressed mice did not induce autoantibodies but still caused myocarditis (Neu et al. 1990). How myosin can trigger myocarditis in these immunosuppressed mice is difficult to envisage. Moreover, passive transfer of a high-titer anti-myosin antibody preparation failed to induce myocarditis (Neu et al. 1990). Because the fine specificity of the different anti-myosin Igs has not been addressed in most of those studies, they are difficult to compare. Myosin is a very large molecule and it is possible that the myosin determinant(s) recognized by the different sera are not identical.

Some authors believe that other mechanisms than molecular mimicry can explain myosin autoreactivity (see Benoist and Mathis 2001; Engman and Leon 2002; Kierszenbaum 2003). They feel that mimicry is less likely to be occurring than Ag release due to myocardial damage leading to expansion of normally tolerant myosin-reactive T cells, particularly because myosin autoimmunity is seen in myocarditis associated with other insults. Thus anti-myosin antibodies are induced in patients with heart disease unrelated to *T. cruzi* infection such as viral myocarditis, myocardial infarction, coronary artery bypass and heart valve surgery, among others (de Scheerder et al. 1989; Fedoseyeva et al. 1999; Nomura et al. 1994). B cell anti-myosin response seems to be mainly responsible for pathology in other heart infections, induced by Coxsackie B3 viral infection (Rose and Hill 1996) or by bacteria (Cunningham 2004). In this regard, it is worth mentioning that peptides of CMhc, a cytoplasmic protein, are associated with MHC class II molecules on APCs even in normal mouse myocardium (Smith and Allen 1992) and MHC class II molecules are increased in the heart of *T. cruzi*-infected patients and animals. Cardiomyocyte damage caused either by parasite replication in the heart or by inflammation may release self-Ags, leading to the induction of anti-heart antibodies rather than anti-cross-reactive *T. cruzi* Ags. Thus it could be likely that the initial heart tissue destruction resulting from infection could induce anti-myosin immunity in Chagas' heart disease, being thus the effect and not the cause of the pathology. Alternatively, is possible that although several pathogens may share the ability to destroy the heart they may have different cross-reactive epitopes with heart proteins (myosin). Thus it is possible that the trigger is the combination of pathogen and damage together, although the fine specificity of the autoreactive response against myosin will be different for each heart pathogen.

In summary, before suggesting a possible role for anti-myosin immunity in Chagas' heart disease, some questions need to be fully addressed: (1) Is the damage during *T. cruzi* infection different from heart tissue injury of a different etiology? (2) Do anti-myosin antibodies truly contribute to chagasic pathology? (3) If anti-myosin antibodies appeared after the occurrence of tissue damage, would they aggravate the pathology by mediating the destruction of intact cardiomyocytes?

5.1.2
Ribosomal Proteins

Another set of autoantigens which have been involved in CCC pathology are ribosomal proteins. Anti-ribosomal P protein antibodies were detected in the serum of chagasic patients and their titer associated with the degree of myocarditis, suggesting a correlation between the appearance of these antibodies and heart pathology (Levin et al. 1990, 1989; Skeiky et al. 1992). By screening a *T. cruzi* expression cDNA library with such sera, some DNA clones were identified. One of the clones, termed JL5, codified for a *T. cruzi* ribosomal protein, TcP2L, and showed sequence homology with human P ribosomal proteins. The homology was between the EDDDMGFGLFD region of Tc2PL and the SD(D/E)DMGFGLFD sequence present in the C-terminal region of human P ribosomal protein (R13 epitope) which was responsible for the cross-reactivity in chagasic serum (Table 3). However, reactivity with ribosomal proteins is also found in some patients with systemic lupus erythematosus (SLE); approximately 15% of SLE patients have autoantibodies to a shared epitope (H13) located in the C-terminal regions of the ribosomal proteins, P0, P1, and P2 (Elkon et al. 1986). However, antibodies against ribosomal proteins from CCC and SLE patients show differential recognition. Thus sera from patients with chronic Chagas' heart disease have been shown to contain relatively high levels of anti-R13 but low levels of anti-H13 antibody (Lopez Bergami et al. 1997), whereas both titers are comparable in SLE sera (Kaplan et al. 1997, 1993). Despite this positive correlation between molecular mimicry and pathology, some discrepancies exist. First, attempts to link anti-R13 reactivity by ELISA in the sera with the symptomatology in chronic or asymptomatic patients failed to find a significant correlation. Thus 60% and 49%, of chronic and asymptomatic sera, respectively, displayed reactivity with R13 but varied significantly depending on the geographical origin of the patients (Aznar et al. 1995). Moreover, no correlation between anti-R13 reactivity and cardiomyopathy was found in a group of 14 patients from whom endomyocardial biopsies and blood samples were taken at the same time. Furthermore, mice immunized with TcP2L developed antibodies against the cross-reactive epitope, as well as many others, in contrast with the fine specificity of antibodies obtained from infected mice (Sepulveda et al. 2000).

On the other hand, some evidence indicates that those anti-P ribosomal antibodies could be pathogenic. Thus purified IgG, reactive with the C-terminus epitope of *T. cruzi* ribosomal P protein, caused a chronotropic alteration in primary rat cardiomyocytes through selective stimulation of β1-adrenergic receptors (Elies et al. 1996; Ferrari et al. 1995). However, in this case, the relevant cross-reactive epitope included the AESDE amino acid sequence from the second extracellular loop of the human β1-adrenergic receptor, which is homologous to the internal AESEE sequence of TcP0 (Table 3) (Ferrari et al. 1995). Moreover, passive transfer of a mAb against R13, which cross-reacts with the human β1-adrenergic receptor, had a chronotropic effect on cultured rat cardiomyocytes (Mahler et al. 2001). Mice immunized with P0 *T. cruzi* ribosomal protein develop electrocardiographic alterations late after immunization, when the titer of antibodies is extremely high, similar to those in chagasic animals but not identical to the complex response of chronic *T. cruzi* infection (Lopez Bergami et al. 2001). In contrast, those hyperimmunized with TcP2L died at an earlier time and did not show heart inflammation.

Sera from chagasic patients also contain IgG antibodies which immunoprecipitated human M2 muscarinic cholinergic receptor molecules and which were able to activate them, having an agonist effect on cardiomyocytes and causing partial desensitization (Leiros et al. 1997). The original stimulus for the formation of these antibodies was not ascertained and whether they could cause heart dysfunctions of the types seen in chagasic patients remains an open question.

5.1.3
Cha

We have described an autoantigen, Cha, a mammalian transcription factor which is recognized by almost all chagasic sera and by sera from *T. cruzi*-infected mice (Girones et al. 2001b). This Ag was isolated by screening of a library with seven CCC sera and has two regions of homology with *T. cruzi*, one with in an expressed sequence tag of the parasite (TENU2845) and another with SAPA, the Ag shed in the acute phase of *T. cruzi* infections (Table 3) (Cazzulo and Frasch 1992; Pollevick et al. 1993). Interestingly, we found that the two epitopes, named R1 and R3, are recognized by T and B cells, respectively, both having significant sequence homology. Very interestingly, there is a strong association of anti-Cha (R3) antibodies and pathology. Thus the titer of the sera from chagasic patients against R3 increases with symptomatology and decreases with treatment (Girones et al. 2001a). However, we have not determined yet whether anti-R3 antibodies have any effect on pathology of the disease. Future experiments will focus on this. Our hypothesis is that these antibodies arise during infection by cooperation of Cha-specific B cells with T cells of different specificity (Fig. 2).

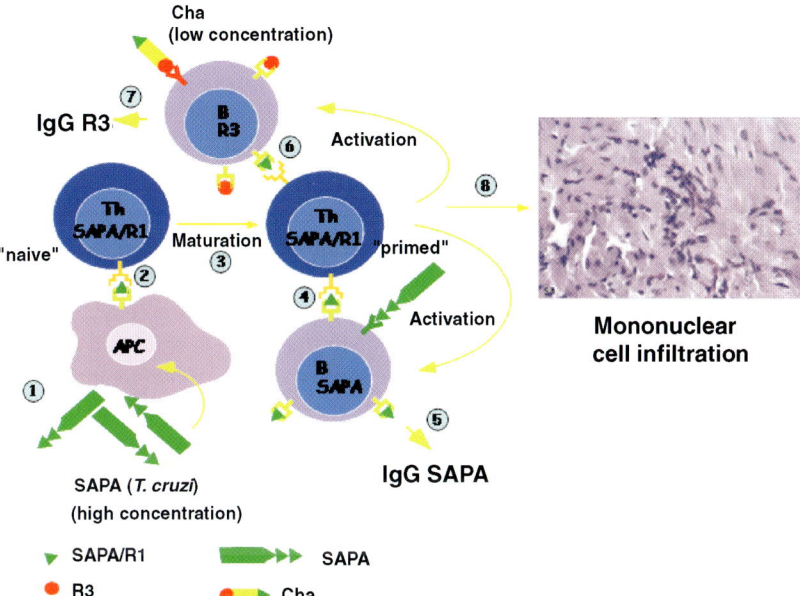

Fig. 2 Generation of anti Cha T/B cell responses. *T. cruzi* infection causes the secretion of parasite Ags to the medium and lyses host's cells, triggering release of self Ags. In particular, during *T. cruzi* infection SAPA Ag is released to the extracellular environment and is taken up by macrophages (*1*). There SAPA is processed intracellularly and presented to naïve T cells through MHC Class II molecules (*2*). These T cells undergo maturation and develop into primed effector T cells specific for SAPA and the cross-reactive epitope R1 of Cha (*3*). Interaction of SAPA/R1 T cells with B cells of the same specificity (*4*) triggers anti-SAPA antibody production (*5*), which is observed during infection. However, the Cha Ag epitopes can be presented on the surface of B cells by MHC Class II molecules by two possible mechanisms: (a) The Cha epitopes can be naturally presented on B cells and (b) the Cha epitopes can be released during infection due to lysis of infected cells. Then, SAPA/R1 T cells can interact with B cells that present the R1 cross-reactive epitope of Cha (*6*) and trigger anti-Cha(R3) antibodies of different specificity (*7*). On the other hand, SAPA/R1 T cells are able to induce inflammatory infiltrates and damage in hearts of recipient mice through cytokines and/or activation of CD8 T cells (*8*)

5.2
Autoreactive T Cells

Perhaps the best evidence supporting a role for autoantigen-specific autoimmunity in disease pathogenesis derives from studies on T cell-mediated immunity in mice. Ribeiro-Dos-Santos et al. have reported that a $CD4^+$ T cell line obtained from a chronic chagasic mouse consisting of approximately 95% $CD4^+$ T cells proliferated in response to either a crude *T. cruzi* Ag preparation or heart tissue extracts from different animal species (Ribeiro-Dos-Santos et al. 2001). In culture, this cell line arrests the beating of fetal heart cells and, more importantly, induces myocarditis in immunized mice and promotes rejection of transplanted normal hearts in the absence of *T. cruzi* (Ribeiro-Dos-Santos et al. 2001). The requirement of the parasite to cause rejection in mice transplanted with T cells from infected mice has been also widely debated (Cunha-Neto et al. 1995; dos Santos et al. 1992; Ribeiro-Dos-Santos et al. 2001; Tarleton et al. 1997). Thus rejection of syngeneic transplanted hearts in chronically infected mice has been shown to take place either in the absence (dos Santos et al. 1992) or in the presence (Tarleton et al., 1997) of the parasite. These differences may be due to the different mice and parasite strain combinations used, and when the presence of the parasite is required for rejection, inflammation and not *T. cruzi* replication may be necessary to provide the necessary adjuvant effect to trigger autoreactivity and could be the rejection-inducing agent in the implanted hearts.

Besides proposing that B cell cross-reactivity against myosin is involved in pathogenesis, Cunha-Neto et al. have also proposed that myosin cross-reactive T lymphocytes infiltrating heart tissue lesions are also involved in chronic chagasic heart tissue lesions (Cunha-Neto et al. 1996, 1995). These T cells are also activated by CMhc cross-reactive *T. cruzi* Ag B13 as in B cells (Cuhna-Neto 2000; Cunha-Neto et al. 1996) (Table 3). Thus T cells from chagasic patients with overt heart disease or asymptomatic patients responded to in vitro stimulation with B13 with increased IFN-γ and reduced IL-4 production, suggesting a Th1-type cytokine profile (Cunha-Neto and Kalil 2001; Cunha-Neto et al. 1998). Those authors proposed that heart damage in CCC could be secondary to the release of inflammatory cytokines and a DTH process initiated by B13. However, the assumption that pathology arises from molecular mimicry between B13 *T. cruzi* and CMhc has been challenged by other authors because T cell autoreactivity against B13 was shown to exist not only in CCC but also in asymptomatic patients and in other cardiopathies (Kierszenbaum 2003). Moreover, both the level of the response to B13 and the cytokine production profile of lymphocytes from asymptomatic chagasic patients were similar to those of T cells from patients with overt heart disease (Cunha-Neto and Kalil 2001).

It is noteworthy that immunological tolerance to heart Ags induced in mice by heart Ag administration and anti-CD4 antibody before their infection by *T. cruzi* resulted in less intense cardiopathy than that in control non-tolerized animals (Pontes-de-Carvalho et al. 2002), which is in favor of an autoimmune pathology. This treatment affects $CD4^+$ responses and not the production of anti-myosin IgG. Although this suggests that the regime to make the mice tolerant was not as effective as expected, at least regarding the humoral response (Th2 mediated), it is becoming increasingly evident that the response involved in heart damage is Th1 mediated. Recently, Leon et al. have described (although in the acute phase) that myosin autoimmunity, while a potentially important inflammatory mechanism in acute and chronic infection, is not essential for cardiac inflammation (Leon et al. 2003), although immunization with a *T. cruzi* extract induced a DTH response against myosin (Leon et al. 2004).

We also studied the T cell response to Cha autoantigen during *T. cruzi* infection. T lymphocytes from *T. cruzi*-infected mice also proliferated to recombinant Cha. More interestingly, transfer of T cells from chronically infected mice to naïve syngeneic mice led to heart infiltration and to production of anti-Cha antibodies, detectable 60 days later (when chronic pathology arises in mice after *T. cruzi* infection) (Girones et al. 2001b). Transferred T cells were almost pure CD3 cells (99%). Consistently, transfer of T cell clones specific for SAPA/R1 cross-reactive epitopes results in heart infiltration in the absence of anti-Cha antibody production (Girones et al., in preparation). Therefore, in some cases the presence of the parasite is not necessary to produce pathology if one transfers activated autoreactive T cells. How this takes place and whether the Cha autoantigen (normally an intracytoplasmic protein) comes to be presented to T cells are under investigation in our laboratory (see Fig. 2 for a hypothetical model). The observed anti-Cha response is likely due to a cooperation of R1-Cha-specific T cells with naïve anti-R3 autoreactive B cells. We believe that Cha autoreactive T cells are responsible for the heart damage, and that Cha autoantibodies are an epiphenomenon secondary to heart tissue destruction. Our results suggest that T cells cooperate with naïve B cells in the animal after heart damage because transfer of T cell clones induces heart infiltration but no anti-Cha antibodies. Although our results suggest that Cha may be involved in pathology, this by no means indicates that Cha would be the only autoantigen involved in the pathology of Chagas' disease.

6
Bystander Activation

As reviewed recently by von Herrath et al. (2003), bystander activation is defined as the activation of autoreactive lymphocytes that do not recognize microbial Ags. This can be mediated through cytokines and/or APCs (TCR-independent bystander activation). However, bystander activation might also require concurrent exposure to the cognate Ag. Ag-specific cells induced by molecular mimicry can be activated by a non-specific stimulus such as other

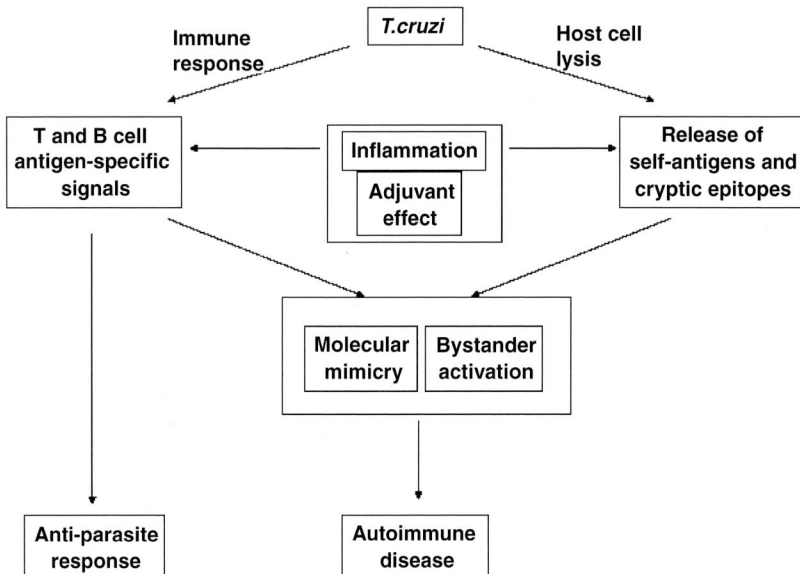

Fig. 3 Diagram of the different mechanisms of induction of pathogenicity by *T. cruzi*. *T. cruzi* induces T and B cell anti-parasite responses which, through molecular mimicry with extracellular Ags or epitopes in Ags normally presented by APCs, can lead to autoimmune disease. *T. cruzi* can lead to secretion of cytokines which mediate some cardiac damage, liberating autoantigens reconized by autoreactive T cells and autoantibodies that further damage the cardiac tissue via bystander activation. Simultaneously parasite replication can induce release of self-antigens, usually intracellular, which contain cryptic epitopes that can be presented by APCs. Also, over-expression of intracellular Ags induced by *T. cruzi* can result in presentation of cryptic epitopes by APCs. If cryptic epitopes are cross-reactive with *T. cruzi* epitopes, then autoimmune disease can arise. *T. cruzi* contains several molecules capable of stimulating the immune system in a non-Ag-specific manner, known as the adjuvant effect, which together with the release of self-antigens and exposure of cryptic epitopes can contribute to sustain a local immune activation known as bystander activation

infections or heart damage, or by adjuvants in experimental settings, to induce autoimmune disease. Regarding *T. cruzi* Ags, both types of bystander activation have been described. *T. cruzi* parasitization of host tissue induces the release of autoantigens (Talvani et al. 2000) and a proinflammatory environment rich in cytokines, nitric oxide and chemokines sufficient to activate autoreactive T cells by lowering the threshold of activation (Fedoseyeva et al. 1999) (see Fig. 3). These cells may then proliferate in response to self-Ag presented on host APC. If this were the case for myosin, aberrant Ag presentation per se would not be necessary, because peptides of cardiac myosin, a cytoplasmic protein, are found complexed with class II MHC molecules on APCs even in normal mouse myocardium (Smith and Allen 1992) and are increased in the heart of infected patients and animals. The anti-self response is initiated and tissue damage may ensue if the response is of sufficient intensity.

7
Parasite Persistence

Despite all the facts mentioned above, several researchers in this field defend the idea that *T. cruzi* persistence in the infected host is solely responsible for the damage in the chronic phase. Tarleton has reviewed all the arguments in favor of the parasite persistence hypothesis to explain the pathogenesis of chronic Chagas' disease in general and of CCC in particular (Tarleton 2001, 2003; Tarleton and Zhang, 1999). Arguments in favor of the idea that disease is linked to parasite presence are supported by the fact that treatments which decrease the parasite burden in the acute phase are associated with a decrease in clinical symptoms (Viotti et al. 1994). Enhancing the efficiency of the anti-parasite response by immunotherapy, gene deletion, or vaccination results in decreased severity of the chronic phase, not exacerbation of disease as predicted by the autoimmune hypothesis (Tarleton 2003). However, this argument cannot be used against autoimmunity because the fine specificity (cross-reactivity?) of those anti-parasite responses was not studied. Effective chemotherapy could also enhance anti-*T. cruzi* immunity in mice (Olivieri et al. 2002). In humans, the link between persistence of *T. cruzi* and clinical disease is also supported by the tissue-specific detection of parasite DNA in the hearts, but not in the esophageal tissue, of individuals with cardiac disease, and vice versa (Jones et al. 1993; Vago et al. 1996). Very recent data in humans show a higher frequency of parasite-specific IFN-γ-producing $CD8^+$ T cells among chronic Chagas' disease patients with mild clinical disease than in those with the most severe form of the disease, supporting a link between the strength and nature of the anti-parasite response and the severity of chronic-stage disease (Laucella et al. 2004). Apparently this supports the parasite persistence hypothesis in opposition to autoimmunity, arguing strongly in favor of the participation of an effective anti-parasite response in preventing disease (Tarleton 2003). Conversely, it has been observed that immunosuppressive treatments correlate with exacerbation of the infection and disease (Ferreira and Borges 2002) although this is not always the case. Thus the use of cyclosporin A has been shown to reactivate parasitemia in several but not all of the heart-transplanted patients. In general, chagasic heart transplants are not rejected or suffer from myocarditis despite the use of immunosuppressive drugs (see Kierszenbaum 2003). These data have been taken as an argument against an autoimmune-based pathology in CCC because transplanted hearts given to patients with the most severe cases of Chagas' heart disease remained essentially undamaged for so many years. However, we need to be cautious because few studies have gone more than 10 years when in a normal infection the pathology of CCC sometimes appears 15–30 years after primary infection. Moreover, if proven true, this mostly discards autoantibodies as the main pathological cause of CCC, but not autoreactive T cells. The same treatment that suppressed alloantigen T cell reactivity may have suppressed autoreactive T cells. So a role for T cells cannot be discarded.

In addition, we have found that autoreactivity in the chronic phase is also linked to parasitemia because the antibody titer and number of reactive T cells against the Cha autoantigen are lower in C57BL/6 (non-susceptible) than in BALB/c (susceptible) mice (Girones et al. 2001b). Moreover, potentially pathogenic anti-Cha autoantibodies also decreased with chemotherapeutic treatment of Chagas' patients. The titer of anti-Cha antibodies, as well as anti-*T. cruzi* antibodies, decreased in parallel with treatment and increased with symptomatology (Girones et al. 2001a) (Table 4). Thus anti-parasite response, some anti-self responses and pathology seem to go together. This poses a word

Table 4 Myocarditis and antibody responses in chagasic patients increase with symptomatology and decrease with treatment

Chagasic patients	Anti-Cha antibodies	Anti-*T. cruzi* antibodies	Myocarditis
Symptomatic	+++	+++	+++
Asymptomatic untreated	++	++	–
Asymptomatic treated	+	+	–

The presence or absence of myocarditis was given by clinical histories of patients. Antibody response was taken from Girones et al. 2001a (OD 450 nm<0.3, [+]; OD 450 nm between 0.3 and 1.0, [++]; OD 450 nm<1.0, [+++]).

of caution in interpreting some clinical data when not all aspects of the problem are measured. Those results may be interpreted in very different ways: (a) the parasite is the only cause of the disease and anti-parasite and anti-self responses are direct consequences of parasite replication, (b) pathology may be caused by the anti-*T. cruzi* response or (c) the parasite is the trigger of autoimmune response which is the effector mechanism.

The presence of *T. cruzi* in the chronic phase of the disease was already observed in early descriptions (Vianna 1911) and was documented subsequently by other authors (Almeida et al. 1984; Teixeira Vde et al. 1993). With more sensitive techniques such as polymerase chain reaction (PCR), the parasite (more properly parasite DNA) is commonly detected in chronic patients (reviewed in Higuchi Mde et al. 2003). Recent immunohistochemistry studies have demonstrated higher frequencies of *T. cruzi* Ags, reaching 100% of hearts from chronic chagasic patients who died due to heart failure when several samples of the myocardium were analyzed (Higuchi 1993; Palomino 2000). Many previous failures to detect parasite Ags in biopsy material from patients in the chronic phase have been attributed to the fact that it seems necessary to examine several different sections of the heart to detect the parasite in this phase of the disease (Higuchi Mde et al. 2003). Using a mouse strain which develops chagasic cardiomyopathy when infected with a highly virulent *T. cruzi* strain, amastigotes were detected in myocytes through the chronic phase, although their numbers were low and much lower than in the acute phase (Guarner et al. 2001). A general finding not always acknowledged by the supporters of the parasite persistence hypothesis is that there is no direct correlation between the sites of parasite detection and heart damage, and also no correlation between the levels of parasites (for example, as detected by PCR) and clinical findings (Monteon-Padilla et al. 2001). However, a significant association between the presence of *T. cruzi* Ags in the heart and severe or moderate inflammation was observed both in humans (Higuchi Mde et al., 2003) and in animal models of the disease (Buckner et al. 1999). However, the number of parasites was low in relation to the intensity of the myocarditis and whole myocardial fibers containing parasites did not elicit inflammation (Higuchi Mde et al. 2003). This suggests two possibilities: exuberant host reactions to the few remaining parasites, either immune mediated or not, or autoimmune-induced inflammation. Parasite Ags probably work as a trigger response against the myocardial fibers. In addition, it is plausible that some lesions lack parasites or parasite Ags because of the effective clearance of parasites from the site by an effective anti-parasite immune response, thus preventing observation of an exact correlation. However, this is difficult to reconcile with the fact that a strong anti-parasite immune response results in decreased symptoms (Laucella et al. 2004).

Thus parasites are somehow present in the chronic phase, but what one ought to know is whether relevant parasite Ags persist and are presented by APCs to T cells. No matter the Ag recognized, Ag-specific T cells must be stimulated to become effector cells (helper, cytotoxic or other). For this, the Ag needs to be presented. Although some APCs could be very efficient in presenting Ags, it is rather unlikely that there are enough parasite Ags to continuously support chronic T cell stimulation.

Recently, it has been shown that *T. cruzi* kinetoplast DNA is able to integrate into human and other mammalian cell genomes and was transmitted to the descendants (Nitz et al. 2004). This has important implications not only for the detection of parasite mentioned above (some based in kinetoplast DNA) but also for pathology, because *T. cruzi* kinetoplast Ag could be continuously presented and may continuously trigger a response to those Ags of the parasite, thus killing normal cells.

8
Coexistence of Parasite Persistence and Autoimmunity

We think that because cardiac myosin autoimmunity develops in the acute phase, when there is lysis of cardiac myocytes and easily detectable parasites, it is very likely that the two processes, bystander damage and molecular mimicry, co-exist until the chronic phase, where damage is produced via effector cells recognizing cross-reactive *T. cruzi*/autoantigen through molecular mimicry.

Thus we propose that the parasite is the trigger which activates some T cells (autoantigen/cross-reactive parasite Ag). Once they are activated, they secrete inflammatory cytokines which mediate some cardiac damage. This liberates autoantigen which is also recognized by some other autoreactive T cells and autoantibodies which further damage the cardiac tissue via bystander activation. This is like a vicious cycle triggered by parasite Ags but fueled by cross-reactive autoantigens and implies that purely parasite-specific T cells may cause very little cardiac damage. This also involves two of the proposed pathogenic mechanisms: bystander damage and molecular mimicry. *T. cruzi* might also function as an adjuvant for an immunological cross-reaction between common parasitic and myocardial fiber Ags, resulting in severe lymphocytic myocarditis (see Fig. 3).

Thus parasites are necessary to trigger autoantibodies and autoreactive T cells and may be necessary to maintain them in the chronic phase. Altogether, we believe that active *T. cruzi* infection is necessary to trigger the autoimmune process, most likely through autoreactive T cells, which once induced can produce the cardiac pathology.

Obviously, the elucidation of the mechanisms of pathogenesis in Chagas' disease may have implications for vaccination and therapy. If autoimmunity by molecular mimicry is responsible, anti-*T. cruzi* chemotherapy would not necessarily suppress pathogenic autoimmune responses initially elicited by parasite Ags and subsequently boosted by host tissue Ags. Also, in the search for protective vaccine we should discard *T. cruzi* Ags that elicit pathogenic anti-self responses.

9
Final Remarks

As mentioned above, several criteria, put originally forth in the *T. cruzi* field by Kierszenbaum 1986 and more broadly by Benoist et al. (Benoist and Mathis, 2001) must be met to consider a disease as caused by molecular mimicry (see Table 2). In *T. cruzi* infection, the first three conditions have been clearly demonstrated, and this has allowed the identification of several candidate autoantigens. If there were a unique cross-reactive Ag, infection with genetically deficient parasites lacking the inducing Ag, or infection of knockout mice lacking the cross-reactive autoantigen, would prevent the disease. However, as multiple autoantigens seem to be involved in the pathology of Chagas' disease, such experiments are very difficult to perform, and therefore the fourth criterion has not been demonstrated yet.

The fifth criterion is considered to be the decisive test of the concept of autoimmunity.

In most publications about autoimmunity in Chagas' disease the putative causes are either autoantibodies or autoreactive T cells originated by molecular mimicry between parasite and host Ags. Nevertheless, evidence for the mediation of cross-reactive antibodies or T cells in pathology is still far from settled. Moreover, most of the data come from experimental *T. cruzi* infection, and an additional problem is the extrapolation of the results to the human model which is more difficult to study.

One way to determine the pathological effect of autoreactive T or B cells would be to immunize mice with cross-reactive Ags to see whether this induces pathology. However, immunization with an autoantigen (injected together with adjuvants and via different routes than natural infection) may not reflect the way the autoantigen is presented during natural infection and may elicit hyperimmune responses, tolerance or regulatory T cells which may suppress autoimmunity. An alternative approach is the transfer of putative autoreactive T cells from chronically infected mice specific for a given autoantigen. Either immunization with or transfer of T cells specific for autoantigens may answer some of these questions and determine which of the candidates are really relevant for pathology. In this respect, the presence of autoreactive T cells against Cha proteins shown in our experiment with Cha autoantigen is the closest to this. Recently, an interesting observation was made by von Herrath et al. (2003), proposed that autoimmune diseases could be induced and exacerbated by many different microbial infections. Their hypothesis is that after infection there is exposure to self, foreign and environmental agents. After clearance of infection, the inflammatory response drops, but when there are additional infections the threshold for autoimmunity is reached and autoaggressive T cells expand and develop.

On the other hand, the parasite persistence hypothesis is based on the fact that *T. cruzi* persists in the chronic phase of Chagas' disease and that treatment against the parasite results in a decrease of the severity of the disease. There are also some questions that need to be fully addressed: (1) Why do lesions develop primarily in the heart and not at other sites of parasite persistence? (2) Why does parasite burden not always correlate with disease severity? A demonstration of these hypotheses is also difficult to perform, because one ought to separate the components of the immune response, self and anti-self during infection. However, we think that things are not so easy, because co-existence of self and non-self Ags would enhance the immune response against both, being always triggered by the parasite.

Acknowledgements The experimental work of the authors mentioned in this manuscript has been supported by grants from: Ministerio de Ciencia y Tecnologia, Red RICET, Fondo de Investigaciones Sanitarias, Comunidad Autonoma de Madrid and Fundacion Ramon Areces. We thank Gloria Escribano for technical assistance in the preparation of this manuscript.

References

Abel, LC, Kalil, J, Cunha Neto, E (1997) Molecular mimicry between cardiac myosin and *Trypanosoma cruzi* antigen B13: identification of a B13-driven human T cell clone that recognizes cardiac myosin. Braz J Med Biol Res 30:1305–1308

Acosta, AM, Santos-Buch, CA (1985) Autoimmune myocarditis induced by *Trypanosoma cruzi*. Circulation 71:1255–1261

Aliberti, JC, Cardoso, MA, Martins, GA, Gazzinelli, RT, Vieira, LQ, Silva, JS (1996) Interleukin-12 mediates resistance to *Trypanosoma cruzi* in mice and is produced by murine macrophages in response to live trypomastigotes. Infect Immun 64:1961–1967

Almeida, HO, Teixeira, VP, Gobbi, H, Rocha, A, Brandao, MC (1984) [Inflammation associated with cardiac muscle cells parasitized by *Trypanosoma cruzi*, in chronic Chagas' disease patients]. Arq Bras Cardiol 42:183–186

Andrade, ZA, Andrade, SG (1955) The pathology of Chagas' disease. (cardiac chronic form). Bol Fund G Moniz 6:1–53

Aznar, C, Lopez-Bergami, P, Brandariz, S, Mariette, C, Liegeard, P, Alves, MD, Barreiro, EL, Carrasco, R, Lafon, S, Kaplan, D, et al. (1995) Prevalence of anti-R-13 antibodies in human *Trypanosoma cruzi* infection. FEMS Immunol Med Microbiol 12:231–238

Ben Younes-Chennoufi, A, Hontebeyrie-Joskowicz, M, Tricottet, V, Eisen, H, Reynes, M, Said, G (1988) Persistence of *Trypanosoma cruzi* antigens in the inflammatory lesions of chronically infected mice. Trans R Soc Trop Med Hyg 82:77–83

Benoist, C, Mathis, D (2001) Autoimmunity provoked by infection: how good is the case for T cell epitope mimicry? Nat Immunol 2:797–801

Benvenuti, LA, Higuchi, ML, Reis, MM (2000) Upregulation of adhesion molecules and class I HLA in the myocardium of chronic chagasic cardiomyopathy and heart allograft rejection, but not in dilated cardiomyopathy. Cardiovasc Pathol 9:111–117

Buckner, FS, Wilson, AJ, Van Voorhis, WC (1999) Detection of live *Trypanosoma cruzi* in tissues of infected mice by using histochemical stain for beta-galactosidase. Infect Immun 67:403–409

Burleigh, BA, Andrews, NW (1998) Signaling and host cell invasion by *Trypanosoma cruzi*. Curr Opin Microbiol 1:461–465

Carrasco Guerra, HA, Palacios-Pru, E, Dagert de Scorza, C, Molina, C, Inglessis, G, Mendoza, RV (1987) Clinical, histochemical, and ultrastructural correlation in septal endomyocardial biopsies from chronic chagasic patients: detection of early myocardial damage. Am Heart J 113:716–724

Castanos-Velez, E, Maerlan, S, Osorio, LM, Aberg, F, Biberfeld, P, Orn, A, Rottenberg, ME (1998) *Trypanosoma cruzi* infection in tumor necrosis factor receptor p55-deficient mice. Infect Immun 66:2960–2968

Cazzulo, JJ, Frasch, AC (1992) SAPA/trans-sialidase and cruzipain: two antigens from *Trypanosoma cruzi* contain immunodominant but enzymatically inactive domains. FASEB J 6:3259–3264

Chagas C (1909) Nova tripanozomiaze humana. Estudos sobre a morfolojia e o ciclo evolutivo do *Schitrypanum cruzi* n. gen., n. sp. Ajente etiolojico de nova entidade morbida do homen. Mem. Inst. Oswaldo Cruz 1:159–219

Cossio, PM, Bustuoabad, O, Paterno, E, Iotti, R, Casanova, MB, Podesta, MR, Bolomo, N, Arana, RM, de Pasqualini, CD (1984) Experimental myocarditis induced in Swiss mice by homologous heart immunization resembles chronic experimental Chagas' heart disease. Clin Immunol Immunopathol 33:165–175

Cossio, PM, Diez, C, Szarfman, A, Kreutzer, E, Candiolo, B, Arana, RM (1974a) Chagasic cardiopathy. Demonstration of a serum gamma globulin factor which reacts with endocardium and vascular structures. Circulation 49:13–21

Cossio, PM, Laguens, RP, Diez, C, Szarfman, A, Segal, A, Arana, RM (1974b) Chagasic cardiopathy. Antibodies reacting with plasma membrane of striated muscle and endothelial cells. Circulation 50:1252–1259

Cuhna-Neto, EaK, J. (2000) Molecular mimicry and Chagas' disease. Microbes and Autoimmunity ASM Press 245–257

Cunha-Neto, E, Coelho, V, Guilherme, L, Fiorelli, A, Stolf, N, Kalil, J (1996) Autoimmunity in Chagas' disease. Identification of cardiac myosin-B13 *Trypanosoma cruzi* protein crossreactive T cell clones in heart lesions of a chronic Chagas' cardiomyopathy patient. J Clin Invest 98:1709–1712

Cunha-Neto, E, Duranti, M, Gruber, A, Zingales, B, De Messias, I, Stolf, N, Bellotti, G, Patarroyo, ME, Pilleggi, F, Kalil, J (1995) Autoimmunity in Chagas disease cardiopathy: biological relevance of a cardiac myosin-specific epitope crossreactive to an immunodominant *Trypanosoma cruzi* antigen. Proc Natl Acad Sci U S A 92:3541–3545

Cunha-Neto, E, Kalil, J (2001) Heart-infiltrating and peripheral T cells in the pathogenesis of human Chagas' disease cardiomyopathy. Autoimmunity 34:187–192

Cunha-Neto, E, Kei, L, Morand, A, Gonçalves, S, Kalil, J. (2004). Autoimmunity in Chagas disease, pp. 449–466. Elsevier.

Cunha-Neto, E, Moliterno, R, Coelho, V, Guilherme, L, Bocchi, E, Higuchi Mde, L, Stolf, N, Pileggi, F, Steinman, L, Kalil, J (1994) Restricted heterogeneity of T cell receptor variable alpha chain transcripts in hearts of Chagas' disease cardiomyopathy patients. Parasite Immunol 16:171–179

Cunha-Neto, E, Rizzo, LV, Albuquerque, F, Abel, L, Guilherme, L, Bocchi, E, Bacal, F, Carrara, D, Ianni, B, Mady, C, Kalil, J (1998) Cytokine production profile of heart-infiltrating T cells in Chagas' disease cardiomyopathy. Braz J Med Biol Res 31:133–137

Cunningham, MW (2004) T cell mimicry in inflammatory heart disease. Mol Immunol 40:1121–1127

Davila, DF, Donis, JH, Torres, A, Gottberg, CF, Rossell, O (1991) Cardiac parasympathetic innervation in Chagas' heart disease. Med Hypotheses 35:80–84

Davila, DF, Rossell, O, de Bellabarba, GA (2002) Pathogenesis of chronic chagas heart disease: parasite persistence and autoimmune responses versus cardiac remodelling and neurohormonal activation. Int J Parasitol 32:107–109

de Scheerder, IK, de Buyzere, ML, Delanghe, JR, Clement, DL, Wieme, RJ (1989) Anti-myosin humoral immune response following cardiac injury. Autoimmunity 4:51–58

Dias, E, Laranja, FS, Miranda, A, Nobrega, G (1956) Chagas' disease; a clinical, epidemiologic, and pathologic study. Circulation 14:1035–1060

dos Santos, PV, Roffe, E, Santiago, HC, Torres, RA, Marino, AP, Paiva, CN, Silva, AA, Gazzinelli, RT, Lannes-Vieira, J (2001) Prevalence of CD8($^+$)alpha beta T cells in *Trypanosoma cruzi*-elicited myocarditis is associated with acquisition of CD62L(Low)LFA-1(High)VLA-4(High) activation phenotype and expression of IFN-gamma-inducible adhesion and chemoattractant molecules. Microbes Infect 3:971–984

dos Santos, RR, Rossi, MA, Laus, JL, Silva, JS, Savino, W, Mengel, J (1992) Anti-CD4 abrogates rejection and reestablishes long-term tolerance to syngeneic newborn hearts grafted in mice chronically infected with *Trypanosoma cruzi*. J Exp Med 175:29–39

Eisen, H, Kahn, S (1991) Mimicry in *Trypanosoma cruzi*: fantasy and reality. Curr Opin Immunol 3:507–510

Elies, R, Ferrari, I, Wallukat, G, Lebesgue, D, Chiale, P, Elizari, M, Rosenbaum, M, Hoebeke, J, Levin, MJ (1996) Structural and functional analysis of the B cell epitopes recognized by anti-receptor autoantibodies in patients with Chagas' disease. J Immunol 157:4203–4211

Elkon, K, Skelly, S, Parnassa, A, Moller, W, Danho, W, Weissbach, H, Brot, N (1986) Identification and chemical synthesis of a ribosomal protein antigenic determinant in systemic lupus erythematosus. Proc Natl Acad Sci U S A 83:7419–7423

Engman, DM, Leon, JS (2002) Pathogenesis of Chagas heart disease: role of autoimmunity. Acta Trop 81:123–132

Factor, SM, Cho, S, Wittner, M, Tanowitz, H (1985) Abnormalities of the coronary microcirculation in acute murine Chagas' disease. Am J Trop Med Hyg 34:246–253

Fedoseyeva, EV, Zhang, F, Orr, PL, Levin, D, Buncke, HJ, Benichou, G (1999) De novo autoimmunity to cardiac myosin after heart transplantation and its contribution to the rejection process. J Immunol 162:6836–6842

Fernandez, MA, Munoz-Fernandez, MA, Fresno, M (1993) Involvement of beta 1 integrins in the binding and entry of *Trypanosoma cruzi* into human macrophages. Eur J Immunol 23:552–557

Ferrari, I, Levin, MJ, Wallukat, G, Elies, R, Lebesgue, D, Chiale, P, Elizari, M, Rosenbaum, M, Hoebeke, J (1995) Molecular mimicry between the immunodominant ribosomal protein P0 of *Trypanosoma cruzi* and a functional epitope on the human beta 1-adrenergic receptor. J Exp Med 182:59–65

Ferreira, MS, Borges, AS (2002) Some aspects of protozoan infections in immunocompromised patients—a review. Mem Inst Oswaldo Cruz 97:443–457

Fourneau, JM, Bach, JM, van Endert, PM, Bach, JF (2004) The elusive case for a role of mimicry in autoimmune diseases. Mol Immunol 40:1095–1102

Fresno, M, Kopf, M, Rivas, L (1997) Cytokines and infectious diseases. Immunol Today 18:56–58

Gazzinelli, RT, Oswald, IP, Hieny, S, James, SL, Sher, A (1992) The microbicidal activity of interferon-gamma-treated macrophages against *Trypanosoma cruzi* involves an L-arginine-dependent, nitrogen oxide-mediated mechanism inhibitable by interleukin-10 and transforming growth factor-beta. Eur J Immunol 22:2501–2506

Giordanengo, L, Fretes, R, Diaz, H, Cano, R, Bacile, A, Vottero-Cima, E, Gea, S (2000a) Cruzipain induces autoimmune response against skeletal muscle and tissue damage in mice. Muscle Nerve 23:1407–1413

Giordanengo, L, Maldonado, C, Rivarola, HW, Iosa, D, Girones, N, Fresno, M, Gea, S (2000b) Induction of antibodies reactive to cardiac myosin and development of heart alterations in cruzipain-immunized mice and their offspring. Eur J Immunol 30:3181–3189

Girones, N, Cuervo, H, Fresno, M (2004) Is there a pathogenic role of autoimmune response in Chagas' disease. Immunología 23:185–199

Girones, N, Rodriguez, CI, Basso, B, Bellon, JM, Resino, S, Munoz-Fernandez, MA, Gea, S, Moretti, E, Fresno, M (2001a) Antibodies to an epitope from the Cha human autoantigen are markers of Chagas' disease. Clin Diagn Lab Immunol 8:1039–1043

Girones, N, Rodriguez, CI, Carrasco-Marin, E, Hernaez, RF, de Rego, JL, Fresno, M (2001b) Dominant T- and B-cell epitopes in an autoantigen linked to Chagas' disease. J Clin Invest 107:985–993

Goni, O, Alcaide, P, Fresno, M (2002) Immunosuppression during acute *Trypanosoma cruzi* infection: involvement of Ly6G (Gr1$^+$)CD11b$^+$ immature myeloid suppressor cells. Int Immunol 14:1125–1134

Gruber, A, Zingales, B (1993) *Trypanosoma cruzi*: characterization of two recombinant antigens with potential application in the diagnosis of Chagas' disease. Exp Parasitol 76:1–12

Guarner, J, Bartlett, J, Zaki, SR, Colley, DG, Grijalva, MJ, Powell, MR (2001) Mouse model for Chagas disease: immunohistochemical distribution of different stages of *Trypanosoma cruzi* in tissues throughout infection. Am J Trop Med Hyg 65:152–158

Henriques-Pons, A, Oliveira, GM, Paiva, MM, Correa, AF, Batista, MM, Bisaggio, RC, Liu, CC, Cotta-De-Almeida, V, Coutinho, CM, Persechini, PM, Araujo-Jorge, TC (2002) Evidence for a perforin-mediated mechanism controlling cardiac inflammation in *Trypanosoma cruzi* infection. Int J Exp Pathol 83:67–79

Higuchi Mde, L, Benvenuti, LA, Martins Reis, M, Metzger, M (2003) Pathophysiology of the heart in Chagas' disease: current status and new developments. Cardiovasc Res 60:96–107

Higuchi, ML, Brito, T., Reis, M. et al. (1993) Correlation between *T. cruzi* and myocardial inflammation in human chronic chagasic myocarditis. Light microscopy and immunohistochemical findings. Cardiovasc Pathol 2:101–106

Higuchi, ML, De Morais, CF, Pereira Barreto, AC, Lopes, EA, Stolf, N, Bellotti, G, Pileggi, F (1987) The role of active myocarditis in the development of heart failure in chronic Chagas' disease: a study based on endomyocardial biopsies. Clin Cardiol 10:665–670

Hoff, R, Teixeira, RS, Carvalho, JS, Mott, KE (1978) *Trypanosoma cruzi* in the cerebrospinal fluid during the acute stage of Chagas' disease. N Engl J Med 298:604–606

Holscher, C, Kohler, G, Muller, U, Mossmann, H, Schaub, GA, Brombacher, F (1998) Defective nitric oxide effector functions lead to extreme susceptibility of *Trypanosoma cruzi*-infected mice deficient in gamma interferon receptor or inducible nitric oxide synthase. Infect Immun 66:1208–1215

Jones, EM, Colley, DG, Tostes, S, Lopes, ER, Vnencak-Jones, CL, McCurley, TL (1993) Amplification of a *Trypanosoma cruzi* DNA sequence from inflammatory lesions in human chagasic cardiomyopathy. Am J Trop Med Hyg 48:348–357

Kalil, J, Cunha-Neto, E (1996) Autoimmunity in Chagas disease cardiomyopathy: Fulfilling the criteria at last? Parasitol Today 12:396–399

Kaplan, D, Ferrari, I, Bergami, PL, Mahler, E, Levitus, G, Chiale, P, Hoebeke, J, Van Regenmortel, MH, Levin, MJ (1997) Antibodies to ribosomal P proteins of *Trypanosoma cruzi* in Chagas disease possess functional autoreactivity with heart tissue and differ from anti-P autoantibodies in lupus. Proc Natl Acad Sci U S A 94:10301–10306

Kaplan, D, Vazquez, M, Lafon, S, Schijman, AG, Levitus, G, Levin, MJ (1993) The chronic presence of the parasite, and anti-P autoimmunity in Chagas disease: the *Trypanosoma cruzi* ribosomal P proteins, and their recognition by the host immune system. Biol Res 26:273–277

Kierszenbaum, F (1986) Autoimmunity in Chagas' disease. J Parasitol 72:201–211

Kierszenbaum, F (1999) Chagas' disease and the autoimmunity hypothesis. Clin Microbiol Rev 12:210–223

Kierszenbaum, F (2003) Views on the autoimmunity hypothesis for Chagas disease pathogenesis. FEMS Immunol Med Microbiol 37:1–11

Kim, EY, Teh, HS (2001) TNF type 2 receptor (p75) lowers the threshold of T cell activation. J Immunol 167:6812–6820

Kirchhoff, LV (1989) Is *Trypanosoma cruzi* a new threat to our blood supply? Ann Intern Med 111:773–775

Kirchhoff, LV (1993) Chagas disease. American trypanosomiasis. Infect Dis Clin North Am 7:487–502

Koberle, F (1961) [Pathology and pathological anatomy of Chagas' disease]. Bol Oficina Sanit Panam 51:404–428

Koberle, F (1970) The causation and importance of nervous lesions in American trypanosomiasis. Bull World Health Organ 42:739–743

Koberle, F, Nador, E (1955) Rev Paul Med 47:643–661

Kumar, S, Tarleton, RL (1998) The relative contribution of antibody production and $CD8^+$ T cell function to immune control of *Trypanosoma cruzi*. Parasite Immunol 20:207–216

Lanzavecchia, A (1995) How can cryptic epitopes trigger autoimmunity? J Exp Med 181:1945–1948

Laucella, SA, Postan, M, Martin, D, Hubby Fralish, B, Albareda, MC, Alvarez, MG, Lococo, B, Barbieri, G, Viotti, RJ, Tarleton, RL (2004) Frequency of interferon-gamma-producing T cells specific for *Trypanosoma cruzi* inversely correlates with disease severity in chronic human Chagas disease. J Infect Dis 189:909–918

Laucella, SA, Segura, EL, Riarte, A, Sosa, ES (1999) Soluble platelet selectin (sP-selectin) and soluble vascular cell adhesion molecule-1 (sVCAM-1) decrease during therapy with benznidazole in children with indeterminate form of Chagas' disease. Clin Exp Immunol 118:423–427

Leiros, CP, Sterin-Borda, L, Borda, ES, Goin, JC, Hosey, MM (1997) Desensitization and sequestration of human m2 muscarinic acetylcholine receptors by autoantibodies from patients with Chagas' disease. J Biol Chem 272:12989–12993

Leon, JS, Daniels, MD, Toriello, KM, Wang, K, Engman, DM (2004) A cardiac myosin-specific autoimmune response is induced by immunization with *Trypanosoma cruzi* proteins. Infect Immun 72:3410–3417

Leon, JS, Engman, DM (2001) Autoimmunity in Chagas heart disease. Int J Parasitol 31:555–561

Leon, JS, Godsel, LM, Wang, K, Engman, DM (2001) Cardiac myosin autoimmunity in acute Chagas' heart disease. Infect Immun 69:5643–5649

Leon, JS, Wang, K, Engman, DM (2003) Myosin autoimmunity is not essential for cardiac inflammation in acute Chagas' disease. J Immunol 171:4271–4277

Levin, MJ (1996) In chronic chagas heart disease, don't forget the parasite. Parasitol. Today 12:415–416

Levin, MJ, Levitus, G, Kerner, N, Lafon, S, Schijman, A, Levy-Yeyati, P, Finkieltein, C, Chiale, P, Schejtman, D, Hontebeyrie-Joskowics, M (1990) Autoantibodies in Chagas' heart disease: possible markers of severe Chagas' heart complaint. Mem Inst Oswaldo Cruz 85:539–543

Levin, MJ, Mesri, E, Benarous, R, Levitus, G, Schijman, A, Levy-Yeyati, P, Chiale, PA, Ruiz, AM, Kahn, A, Rosenbaum, MB, et al. (1989) Identification of major *Trypanosoma cruzi* antigenic determinants in chronic Chagas' heart disease. Am J Trop Med Hyg 41:530–538

Levitus, G, Hontebeyrie-Joskowicz, M, Van Regenmortel, MH, Levin, MJ (1991) Humoral autoimmune response to ribosomal P proteins in chronic Chagas heart disease. Clin Exp Immunol 85:413–417

Lopez Bergami, P, Cabeza Meckert, P, Kaplan, D, Levitus, G, Elias, F, Quintana, F, Van Regenmortel, M, Laguens, R, Levin, MJ (1997) Immunization with recombinant *Trypanosoma cruzi* ribosomal P2beta protein induces changes in the electrocardiogram of immunized mice. FEMS Immunol Med Microbiol 18:75–85

Lopez Bergami, P, Scaglione, J, Levin, MJ (2001) Antibodies against the carboxyl-terminal end of the *Trypanosoma cruzi* ribosomal P proteins are pathogenic. FASEB J 15:2602–2612

Mahler, E, Hoebeke, J, Levin, MJ (2004) Structural and functional complexity of the humoral response against the *Trypanosoma cruzi* ribosomal P2 beta protein in patients with chronic Chagas' heart disease. Clin Exp Immunol 136:527–534

Mahler, E, Sepulveda, P, Jeannequin, O, Liegeard, P, Gounon, P, Wallukat, G, Eftekhari, P, Levin, MJ, Hoebeke, J, Hontebeyrie, M (2001) A monoclonal antibody against the immunodominant epitope of the ribosomal P2beta protein of *Trypanosoma cruzi* interacts with the human beta 1-adrenergic receptor. Eur J Immunol 31:2210–2216

Marino, AP, Azevedo, MI, Lannes-Vieira, J (2003a) Differential expression of adhesion molecules shaping the T-cell subset prevalence during the early phase of autoimmune and *Trypanosoma cruzi*-elicited myocarditis. Mem Inst Oswaldo Cruz 98:945–952

Marino, AP, Silva, AA, Pinho, RT, Lannes-Vieira, J (2003b) *Trypanosoma cruzi* infection: a continuous invader-host cell cross talk with participation of extracellular matrix and adhesion and chemoattractant molecules. Braz J Med Biol Res 36:1121–1133

Martin, D, Tarleton, R (2004) Generation, specificity, and function of CD8$^+$ T cells in *Trypanosoma cruzi* infection. Immunol Rev 201:304–317

Mazza, S (1949) La enfermedad de Chagas en la Rep. Argentina. Mem Inst. Oswaldo Cruz 47:273–288

McCormick, TS, Rowland, EC (1989) *Trypanosoma cruzi*: cross-reactive anti-heart autoantibodies produced during infection in mice. Exp Parasitol 69:393–401

Moncayo, A (1999) Progress towards interruption of transmission of Chagas disease. Mem Inst Oswaldo Cruz 94 Suppl 1:401–404

Monteon-Padilla, V, Hernandez-Becerril, N, Ballinas-Verdugo, MA, Aranda-Fraustro, A, Reyes, PA (2001) Persistence of *Trypanosoma cruzi* in chronic chagasic cardiopathy patients. Arch Med Res 32:39–43

Morris, SA, Tanowitz, HB, Wittner, M, Bilezikian, JP (1990) Pathophysiological insights into the cardiomyopathy of Chagas' disease. Circulation 82:1900–1909

Muñoz-Fernandez, MA, Fernandez, MA, Fresno, M (1992) Synergism between tumor necrosis factor-alpha and interferon-gamma on macrophage activation for the killing of intracellular *Trypanosoma cruzi* through a nitric oxide-dependent mechanism. Eur J Immunol 22:301–307

Neu, N, Ploier, B, Ofner, C (1990) Cardiac myosin-induced myocarditis. Heart autoantibodies are not involved in the induction of the disease. J Immunol 145:4094–4100

Neu, N, Rose, NR, Beisel, KW, Herskowitz, A, Gurri-Glass, G, Craig, SW (1987) Cardiac myosin induces myocarditis in genetically predisposed mice. J Immunol 139:3630–3636

Nitz, N, Gomes, C, de Cassia Rosa, A, D'Souza-Ault, MR, Moreno, F, Lauria-Pires, L, Nascimento, RJ, Teixeira, AR (2004) Heritable integration of kDNA minicircle sequences from *Trypanosoma cruzi* into the avian genome: insights into human Chagas disease. Cell 118:175–186

Nomura, Y, Yoshinaga, M, Haraguchi, T, Oku, S, Noda, T, Miyata, K, Umebayashi, Y, Taira, A (1994) Relationship between the degree of injury at operation and the change in antimyosin antibody titer in the postpericardiotomy syndrome. Pediatr Cardiol 15:116–120

Oldstone, MB (1989) Overview: infectious agents as etiologic triggers of autoimmune disease. Curr Top Microbiol Immunol 145:1–3

Olivieri, BP, Cotta-De-Almeida, V, Araujo-Jorge, T (2002) Benznidazole treatment following acute *Trypanosoma cruzi* infection triggers CD8$^+$ T-cell expansion and promotes resistance to reinfection. Antimicrob Agents Chemother 46:3790–3796

Palomino, AS, Aiello, V.D., Higuchi, M.L. (2000) Systematic mapping of hearts from chronic chagasic patients: the association between the occurrence of histopathological lesions and *Trypanosoma cruzi* antigens. Ann Trop Med Parasitol 6:571–579

Penninger, JM, Bachmaier, K (2000) Review of microbial infections and the immune response to cardiac antigens. J Infect Dis 181 Suppl 3:S498–504

Pereira Barretto, AC, Mady, C, Arteaga-Fernandez, E, Stolf, N, Lopes, EA, Higuchi, ML, Bellotti, G, Pileggi, F (1986) Right ventricular endomyocardial biopsy in chronic Chagas' disease. Am Heart J 111:307–312

Petkova, SB, Huang, H, Factor, SM, Pestell, RG, Bouzahzah, B, Jelicks, LA, Weiss, LM, Douglas, SA, Wittner, M, Tanowitz, HB (2001) The role of endothelin in the pathogenesis of Chagas' disease. Int J Parasitol 31:499–511

Pollevick, GD, Sanchez, DO, Campetella, O, Trombetta, S, Sousa, M, Henriksson, J, Hellman, U, Pettersson, U, Cazzulo, JJ, Frasch, AC (1993) Members of the SAPA/trans-sialidase protein family have identical N-terminal sequences and a putative signal peptide. Mol Biochem Parasitol 59:171–174

Pontes-de-Carvalho, L, Santana, CC, Soares, MB, Oliveira, GG, Cunha-Neto, E, Ribeiro-dos-Santos, R (2002) Experimental chronic Chagas' disease myocarditis is an autoimmune disease preventable by induction of immunological tolerance to myocardial antigens. J Autoimmun 18:131–138

Prata, A (1994) Chagas' disease. Infect Dis Clin North Am 8:61–76

Prata, A (2001) Clinical and epidemiological aspects of Chagas disease. Lancet Infect Dis 1:92–100

Reis, DD, Jones, EM, Tostes, S, Lopes, ER, Chapadeiro, E, Gazzinelli, G, Colley, DG, McCurley, TL (1993) Expression of major histocompatibility complex antigens and adhesion molecules in hearts of patients with chronic Chagas' disease. Am J Trop Med Hyg 49:192–200

Ribeiro-Dos-Santos, R, Mengel, JO, Postol, E, Soares, RA, Ferreira-Fernandez, E, Soares, MB, Pontes-De-Carvalho, LC (2001) A heart-specific $CD4^+$ T-cell line obtained from a chronic chagasic mouse induces carditis in heart-immunized mice and rejection of normal heart transplants in the absence of *Trypanosoma cruzi*. Parasite Immunol 23:93–101

Rose, NR (2001) Infection, mimics, and autoimmune disease. J Clin Invest 107:943–944

Rose, NR, Hill, SL (1996) The pathogenesis of postinfectious myocarditis. Clin Immunol Immunopathol 80:S92–99

Rose, NR, Mackay, IR (2000) Molecular mimicry: a critical look at exemplary instances in human diseases. Cell Mol Life Sci 57:542–551

Rossi, L (1996) Neuropathology of chronic chagasic cardiopathy: A diagnostic reassessment. Cardiovasc Pathol 5:233–239.

Santos-Buch, CA, Teixeira, AR (1974) The immunology of experimental Chagas' disease. 3. Rejection of allogeneic heart cells in vitro. J Exp Med 140:38–53

Sepulveda, P, Liegeard, P, Wallukat, G, Levin, MJ, Hontebeyrie, M (2000) Modulation of cardiocyte functional activity by antibodies against *Trypanosoma cruzi* ribosomal P2 protein C terminus. Infect Immun 68:5114–5119

Silva, JS, Morrissey, PJ, Grabstein, KH, Mohler, KM, Anderson, D, Reed, SG (1992) Interleukin 10 and interferon gamma regulation of experimental *Trypanosoma cruzi* infection. J Exp Med 175:169–174

Skeiky, YA, Benson, DR, Parsons, M, Elkon, KB, Reed, SG (1992) Cloning and expression of *Trypanosoma cruzi* ribosomal protein P0 and epitope analysis of anti-P0 autoantibodies in Chagas' disease patients. J Exp Med 176:201–211

Smith, SC, Allen, PM (1992) Expression of myosin-class II major histocompatibility complexes in the normal myocardium occurs before induction of autoimmune myocarditis. Proc Natl Acad Sci U S A 89:9131–9135

Soares, MB, Pontes-De-Carvalho, L, Ribeiro-Dos-Santos, R (2001) The pathogenesis of Chagas' disease: when autoimmune and parasite-specific immune responses meet. An Acad Bras Cienc 73:547–559

Stauffer, Y, Marguerat, S, Meylan, F, Ucla, C, Sutkowski, N, Huber, B, Pelet, T, Conrad, B (2001) Interferon-alpha-induced endogenous superantigen. A model linking environment and autoimmunity. Immunity 15:591–601

Sterin-Borda, L, Giordanengo, L, Joensen, L, Gea, S (2003) Cruzipain induces autoantibodies against cardiac muscarinic acetylcholine receptors. Functional and pathological implications. Eur J Immunol 33:2459–2468

Takle, GB, Hudson, L (1989) Autoimmunity and Chagas' disease. Curr Top Microbiol Immunol 145:79–92

Talvani, A, Ribeiro, CS, Aliberti, JC, Michailowsky, V, Santos, PV, Murta, SM, Romanha, AJ, Almeida, IC, Farber, J, Lannes-Vieira, J, Silva, JS, Gazzinelli, RT (2000) Kinetics of cytokine gene expression in experimental chagasic cardiomyopathy: tissue parasitism and endogenous IFN-gamma as important determinants of chemokine mRNA expression during infection with *Trypanosoma cruzi*. Microbes Infect 2:851–866

Tanowitz, HB, Kirchhoff, LV, Simon, D, Morris, SA, Weiss, LM, Wittner, M (1992) Chagas' disease. Clin Microbiol Rev 5:400–419

Tarleton, RL (2001) Parasite persistence in the aetiology of Chagas disease. Int J Parasitol 31:550–554

Tarleton, RL (2003) Chagas disease: a role for autoimmunity? Trends Parasitol 19:447–451

Tarleton, RL, Zhang, L (1999) Chagas disease etiology: autoimmunity or parasite persistence? Parasitol Today 15:94–99

Tarleton, RL, Zhang, L, Downs, MO (1997) "Autoimmune rejection" of neonatal heart transplants in experimental Chagas disease is a parasite-specific response to infected host tissue. Proc Natl Acad Sci U S A 94:3932–3937

Teixeira Vde, P, Araujo, MB, dos Reis, MA, dos Reis, L, Silveira, SA, Rodrigues, ML, Franquini Junior, J (1993) Possible role of an adrenal parasite reservoir in the pathogenesis of chronic *Trypanosoma cruzi* myocarditis. Trans R Soc Trop Med Hyg 87:552–554

Torrico, F, Heremans, H, Rivera, MT, Van Marck, E, Billiau, A, Carlier, Y (1991) Endogenous IFN-gamma is required for resistance to acute *Trypanosoma cruzi* infection in mice. J Immunol 146:3626–3632

Vago, AR, Macedo, AM, Adad, SJ, Reis, DD, Correa-Oliveira, R (1996) PCR detection of *Trypanosoma cruzi* DNA in oesophageal tissues of patients with chronic digestive Chagas' disease. Lancet 348:891–892

Vakkila, J, Aysto, S, Saarinen-Pihkala, UM, Sariola, H (2001) Naive $CD4^+$ T cells can be sensitized with IL-7. Scand J Immunol 54:501–505

Van Voorhis, WC, Schlekewy, L, Trong, HL (1991) Molecular mimicry by *Trypanosoma cruzi*: the F1-160 epitope that mimics mammalian nerve can be mapped to a 12-amino acid peptide. Proc Natl Acad Sci U S A 88:5993–5997

Vianna, G (1911) Contribuiçao para o estudo da anatomia patologica da Molestia de Carlos Chagas'. Mem Inst Oswaldo Cruz 3:276–293

Viotti, R, Vigliano, C, Armenti, H, Segura, E (1994) Treatment of chronic Chagas' disease with benznidazole: clinical and serologic evolution of patients with long-term follow-up. Am Heart J 127:151–162

von Herrath, MG, Fujinami, RS, Whitton, JL (2003) Microorganisms and autoimmunity: making the barren field fertile? Nat Rev Microbiol 1:151–157

Wendel, S (1998) Transfusion-transmitted Chagas' disease. Curr Opin Hematol 5:406–411

Wood, JN, Hudson, L, Jessell, TM, Yamamoto, M (1982) A monoclonal antibody defining antigenic determinants on subpopulations of mammalian neurones and *Trypanosoma cruzi* parasites. Nature 296:34–38

Wucherpfennig, KW (2001) Structural basis of molecular mimicry. J Autoimmun 16:293–302

HTLV-1 Induced Molecular Mimicry in Neurological Disease

S. M. Lee · Y. Morcos · H. Jang · J. M. Stuart · M. C. Levin (✉)

Department of Neurology, University of Tennessee Health Sciences Center, Link Building, Room 415, 855 Monroe Avenue, Memphis, TN 38163, USA
mlevin@utmem.edu

1	Background 126
2	The Role of the Immune Response in the Pathogenesis of HAM/TSP 127
3	Experimental Data Indicating a Role for Molecular Mimicry in the Pathogenesis of HAM/TSP 128
4	Conclusions 131

References 133

Abstract As a model for molecular mimicry, we study patients infected with human T-lymphotropic virus type 1 (HTLV-1) who develop a neurological disease called HTLV-1-associated myelopathy/tropical spastic paraparesis (HAM/TSP), a disease with important biological similarities to multiple sclerosis (MS) (Khan et al. 2001; Levin et al. 1998, 2002a; Levin and Jacobson 1997). The study of HAM/TSP, a disease associated with a known environmental agent (HTLV-1), allows for the direct comparison of the infecting agent with host antigens. Neurological disease in HAM/TSP patients is associated with immune responses to HTLV-1-tax (a regulatory and immunodominant protein) and human histocompatibility leukocyte antigen (HLA) DRB1*0101 (Bangham 2000; Jacobson et al. 1990; Jeffery et al. 1999; Lal 1996). Recently, we showed that HAM/TSP patients make antibodies to heterogeneous nuclear ribonuclear protein A1 (hnRNP A1), a neuron-specific autoantigen (Levin et al. 2002a). Monoclonal antibodies to tax cross-reacted with hnRNP A1, indicating molecular mimicry between the two proteins. Infusion of cross-reactive antibodies with an ex vivo system completely inhibited neuronal firing indicative of their pathogenic nature (Kalume et al. 2004; Levin et al. 2002a). These data demonstrate a clear link between chronic viral infection and autoimmune disease of the central nervous system (CNS) in humans and, we believe, in turn will give insight into the pathogenesis of MS.

1
Background

The purpose of this review is to examine the potential role of molecular mimicry in the pathogenesis of human T-lymphotropic virus type 1 ((HTLV-1)-associated myelopathy/tropical spastic paraparesis (HAM/TSP)). Comprehensive reviews on the pathogenic mechanisms of HTLV-1-associated human diseases are available throughout the medical literature (Bangham 2000,, 2003; Barmak et al. 2003; Jacobson 2002; Levin and Jacobson 1997; Nagai and Osame 2003; Osame 2002). Approximately 25 years ago the first human retrovirus, HTLV-1, was isolated (Poeisz et al. 1980). Subsequently, infection with HTLV-1 was shown to cause adult T-cell leukemia (ATL) and HAM/TSP (Gessain et al. 1985; McFarlin and Blattner 1991; Osame et al. 1986; Poeisz et al. 1980; Yoshida et al. 1987). HTLV-1 may infect up to 30% of people in endemic areas and 10–20 million people worldwide (Barmak et al. 2003; Edlich et al. 2000). However, only 1%–5% develop either ATL or HAM/TSP, the remainder being clinically asymptomatic carriers of HTLV-1 (Bangham 2000, 2003; Barmak et al. 2003; Jacobson 2002; Levin and Jacobson 1997; Nagai and Osame 2003; Osame 2002). Why infection with HTLV-1 causes ATL or HAM/TSP in some people while the vast majority of individuals are asymptomatic is largely unknown. Some possible factors that may differentiate the asymptomatic from the diseased state include viral strain, human histocompatibility leukocyte antigen (HLA), viral load, and the immune response (Bangham 2000, 2003; Barmak et al. 2003; Jacobson 2002; Levin and Jacobson 1997; Nagai and Osame 2003; Nagai et al. 1998; Niewiesk et al. 1994; Osame 2002).

Clinically, HAM/TSP is more common in women than men, and age of onset is between 35 and 45 years. People with HAM/TSP develop progressive, spastic paraparesis. Weakness of the lower extremities is due to damage of the corticospinal tract, the major motor pathway of the CNS. Weakness is typically symmetrical and slowly progressive and, over time, may ascend to include the upper extremities. Bladder symptoms are common because of the spinal cord involvement of the disease. Sensory symptoms such as paresthesias also occur, suggesting involvement of the posterior columns of the spinal cord; however, sensory involvement is minor compared to motor dysfunction in these patients (Hollsberg and Hafler 1993; Khan et al. 2001; Levin et al. 1997; Levin and Jacobson 1997; McFarlin and Blattner 1991; Nakagawa et al. 1995).

The study of the neuropathology of HAM/TSP revealed two important features: First, CNS damage correlates strongly with the clinical features of the disease and second, the immune system is involved in the pathogenesis of HAM/TSP. Pathologically, there is severe demyelination and axonal dystrophy of the corticospinal tract and posterior columns throughout the brain and spinal cord. Associated with this CNS damage is a robust immune response that includes damage to the blood-brain barrier, infiltrating lymphocytes, macrophages, immunoglobulins, and local cytokine production (Giraudon et al. 2000; Izumo et al. 2000; Jernigan et al. 2003; Levin et al. 1997; Moore et al. 1989; Romero et al. 2000; Umehara et al., 1998, 2002; Wu et al. 1993). Because of this intense inflammatory response in the CNS, immune mechanisms are thought to play a critical role in the pathogenesis of HAM/TSP.

2
The Role of the Immune Response in the Pathogenesis of HAM/TSP

The mechanism by which CNS damage occurs in HAM/TSP is incompletely understood but provides an excellent model that takes into account the relationship among infection with an environmental agent, genetic background, the host immune response, and potential autoantigens in the pathogenesis of autoimmune disease of the nervous system. There is no experimental evidence that direct infection of the CNS results in neural cell damage (Bangham 2000; Hollsberg and Hafler 1993; Levin and Jacobson 1997; Osame 2002). Instead, several observations support the hypothesis that immune-mediated mechanisms play a crucial role. HAM/TSP patients have higher antibody and cytokine levels in sera and cerebrospinal fluid (CSF) than do patients infected with HTLV-1 who lack neurological symptoms (Levin and Jacobson 1997; Osame et al. 1987). It is the immune response to HTLV-1-*env* and *tax*, two immunodominant proteins, that differentiates patients with HAM/TSP from control populations (Bangham 2000; Goon et al. 2002; Jacobson et al. 1990; Lal et al. 1994; Noraz et al. 1993). Specifically, HAM/TSP patients develop a $CD8^+$ cytotoxic T-lymphocyte (CTL) response specific for the N-terminal of HTLV-1-tax (tax$^{11-19}$ in association with HLA-A2) (Bangham 2000; Elovaara et al. 1993; Jacobson et al. 1990). Whether these CTLs are pathogenic or protective is an area of ongoing investigation. Some data suggest that tax-specific CTLs enter the CNS and cause tissue damage (Jacobson 2002). Other studies suggest that high levels of tax-specific CTLs in association with HLA-A2 protect against the development of HAM/TSP (Bangham 2000; Jeffery et al. 1999). In contrast to HLA-2, which may be protective, HLA-DRB1*0101 was found to double the risk of HAM/TSP (Jeffery et al. 1999). Other studies implicate a role for $CD4^+$ T-helper lymphocytes in the pathogenesis of HAM/TSP. Specifically, $CD4^+$ T-lymphocytes are present in the CNS of HAM/TSP patients early in disease (Levin and Jacobson 1997; Osame 2002). Also, HAM/TSP patients develop $CD4^+$ T-helper lymphocytes specific for *env* and *tax* that secrete increased levels of interferon-γ (IFN-γ) compared to interleukin-4 (IL-4), suggesting a Th1 phenotype (Goon et al. 2002). Antibodies also play a role in the pathogenesis of HAM/TSP (Levin and Jacobson 1997; Osame 2002). HAM/TSP patients have elevated antibody titers to HTLV-1 in sera and CSF and exhibit increased intrathecal synthesis of IgG (Levin and Jacobson 1997; Osame et al. 1987). Some studies suggest that antibody titer is proportional to severity of disease (Levin and Jacobson 1997; Osame et al. 1987). Patients infected with HTLV-1 preferentially react with *env* proteins, which are used to diagnose infection (Lal 1996; Noraz et al. 1993). The IgG response in HAM/TSP patients to tax is to the C terminus ($tax^{316-335}$) (Lal, 1996; Rudolph et al., 1994). Data also indicate that viral load is important in stimulating the immune responses in HAM/TSP because these patients have elevated viral loads of tax (Bangham 2000; Nagai et al. 1998; Saito et al. 2004). Also, HTLV-1-infected patients showed marked immunoreactivity to a number of nuclear and cytoplasmic autoantigens (Muller et al. 1995). These data suggest that a cross-reactive immune response between immunodominant HTLV-1 proteins and a CNS autoantigen may exist and contribute to the pathogenesis of HAM/TSP. However, a specific CNS autoantigen that may act as a target for a cellular or antibody-mediated autoimmune response has not been identified. Our data indicate that there is molecular mimicry between HTLV-1 and hnRNP A1 derived from neurons and that mimicry is likely to be significantly involved in the pathogenesis of HAM/TSP (Levin et al. 1998, 2002a).

3
Experimental Data Indicating a Role for Molecular Mimicry in the Pathogenesis of HAM/TSP

Because HAM/TSP patients develop damage specifically of the CNS, we hypothesized that patients would make antibodies to a CNS antigen and that this immune response would play a role in the pathogenesis of the disease. To test this hypothesis, we isolated IgG from the sera of HAM/TSP and control patients, biotinylated it, and reacted it with normal human tissues, using immunohistochemistry. IgG from HAM/TSP patients, in contrast to seronegative controls, stained CNS neurons (Levin et al. 1998, 2002a). Furthermore, the HAM/TSP IgG did not stain CNS glial cells or sections derived from systemic organs. In similar experiments, a monoclonal antibody to HTLV-1-tax (tax Mab) also stained CNS neurons, but not glial cells (Levin et al. 1998, 2002a). This suggests that molecular mimicry exists between the tax epitope recognized by the Mab and a neuronal autoantigen.

To identify the autoantigen, neurons derived from human brain were purified and the neuronal proteins were separated by two-dimensional gel electrophoresis and transferred to membranes for Western blot using biotinylated HAM/TSP IgG. The HAM/TSP IgG reacted with neuronal proteins with molecular weights of 34,000 and 38,000, pI 9.3 (Levin et al. 2002a). Immunoreactive proteins were dissected from the gels, trypsinized, and analyzed by matrix-assisted laser desorption ionization (MALDI) mass spectroscopy. The protein was identified as hnRNP A1 (Levin et al. 2002a). We then cloned and expressed hnRNP A1. We showed that the molecular weight of hnRNP A1 was identical to that of the neuronal autoantigen and that preincubation of HAM/TSP IgG with hnRNP A1 abolished immunoreactivity to neurons by Western blot, thus proving that the autoantigen is hnRNP A1. Importantly, IgG isolated from 10 of 10 HAM/TSP patients reacted with hnRNP A1, in contrast to 0 of 10 controls. This established hnRNP A1 as an autoantigen associated with the development of HAM/TSP (Levin et al. 2002a).

To confirm that the immune reaction was specific for the CNS, we extracted proteins from human organs and tested them for immunoreactivity with HAM/TSP IgG by Western blot. These data showed that HAM/TSP IgG only reacted with neurons derived from brain and recombinant hnRNP A1. There was no reactivity to proteins isolated from systemic organs (Jernigan et al. 2003). Next, because HAM/TSP patients develop clinical and pathological damage to corticospinal pathways, we hypothesized that HAM/TSP IgG would preferentially react with neurons of this motor system. We separated neurons of the precentral gyrus (motor cortex that contains Betz cells, the neurons of origin of the corticospinal tract) from other cortical areas of normal, HTLV-1 seronegative, human brain. Western blots of pre-central gyrus neurons showed an intense signal with HAM/TSP IgG, in contrast to other brain areas. These observations correlated with immunohistochemical staining with HAM/TSP IgG, in which intense labeling was evident in the pyramidal and Betz cells of the pre-central gyrus compared to neurons of the parietal-occipital lobe (Levin et al. 2002a). Concurrently, we hypothesized that antibody deposition in HAM/TSP autopsy specimens would localize to the corticospinal system. In histological sections derived from the brain of HAM/TSP patients, in situ IgG localized to the corticospinal system, including neurons of the frontal cortex and pre-central gyrus, as well as within corticospinal axons in subcortical white matter, periventricular white matter, posterior limb of the internal capsule, midbrain, pons, and medulla (Jernigan et al. 2003). Also, IgG isolated directly from the brain and CSF of HAM/TSP patients reacted with hnRNP A1 (Jernigan et al. 2003; Levin et al. 2002a). These data indicate that HAM/TSP IgG reactivity is highly specific for neurons and axons of the corticospinal tract, the major site of neurological dysfunction in HAM/TSP patients.

In addition to HAM/TSP IgG, the tax Mab also reacted with hnRNP A1 (Levin et al. 2002a). The epitope of the tax Mab was unknown. Using the Mimotope Multipin system (in which 15-mer peptides are synthesized that represent the 353-amino acid sequence of tax), we mapped the epitope of the tax Mab to the C terminal of tax (tax$^{346-353}$) (Levin et al. 2002b). This region overlaps the antibody immunodominant domain (tax$^{329-353}$) in humans (Lal 1996; Levin et al. 2002b). Preincubation of the tax Mabs with increasing concentrations of the C-terminal peptide (KHFRETEV, tax$^{346-353}$) inhibited antibody binding to tax, hnRNP A1, and CNS neurons (Levin et al. 2002b). These data indicate that there is molecular mimicry between HTLV-1-tax and hnRNP A1, and that the mimicking epitope of tax coincides with the immunodominant domain for IgG in humans.

We also have preliminary data on the hnRNP A1 epitope reactive with sera from HAM/TSP patients. hnRNP A1 is an RNA binding protein that is critical for the transport of mRNA from the nucleus to the cytoplasm and cellular processes (Krecic and Swanson 1999; Nakielny and Dreyfuss 1997; Shyu and Wilkinson 2000). The N-terminal portion of the protein binds RNA at two specific sites known as the RNA binding domains (RBDs). The C terminus includes a sequence known as M9, which is the nuclear localization signal (NLS) and nuclear export signal (NES), the sequence required for transport of hnRNP A1 in and out of the nucleus. We designed primers representing the RBDs and the C terminus of hnRNP A1. Protein fragments representing these sequences were cloned, expressed, separated by gel electrophoresis, transferred to membranes, and used for Western blotting with HAM/TSP IgG. There was intense immunoreactivity to the C terminus of hnRNP A1, but not to the N terminus. We then expressed the M9 sequence and found that HAM/TSP IgG was specific for it compared to other fragments contained within the C-terminal sequence (unpublished observation).

Database analyses showed no exact match between tax and hnRNP A1. This suggests that molecular mimicry between these two proteins is based on immunological cross-reactivity rather than on primary sequence. Because epitope binding is based on three-dimensional structure, these and other studies suggest that molecular mimicry, defined by cellular or antibody-mediated cross-reactivity, has increased biological significance compared to that defined by primary sequence analysis (Albert and Inman 1999; Gran et al. 1999; Oldstone 1998; Wucherpfennig 2002).

Next, we designed experiments to test whether cross-reactive antibodies to HTLV-1-tax and hnRNP A1 were pathogenic to neurons. We used neuronal patch-clamp techniques in which brain slices containing motor cortex were removed from rats and submerged in a recording chamber containing CSF. Antibodies were circulated in the extracellular CSF, and recordings were taken from individual neurons. Under these conditions, HAM/TSP IgG, in concentrations of IgG equal to those in human CSF, inhibited neuronal firing in a concentration-dependent manner. Similarly, the tax Mab and affinity-purified antibodies to hnRNP A1 also completely inhibited neuronal firing. Neither IgG isolated from normal individuals nor a Mab to neurofilament inhibited neuronal firing (Kalume et al. 2004; Levin et al. 2002a). These data indicate that antibodies to HTLV-1-tax and hnRNP A1 are biologically active and that a cross-reactive immune response between HTLV-1-tax and hnRNP A1 is pathogenic to neurons (Kalume et al. 2004; Levin et al. 2002a).

4
Conclusions

How autoimmune disease develops in the CNS is incompletely understood but is related to interactions among several factors including genetic background (such as HLA), environmental agents, autoantigens, and the immune response. One hypothesis that couples infections with autoimmune disease is molecular mimicry (see Fig. 1). We believe that HAM/TSP is an excellent model to test molecular mimicry because it is associated with a specific environmental agent (HTLV-1), HLA (DRB*0101), and a robust immune response to viral antigens and autoantigens (Bangham 2000, 2003; Barmak et al. 2003; Jacobson 2002; Levin and Jacobson 1997; Muller et al. 1995; Nagai and Osame 2003; Osame 2002). Using this model, we determined that HAM/TSP patients develop an antibody response to normal CNS neurons that cross-reacts with HTLV-1-tax. The immunoreactive component of the neuron is hnRNP A1. Importantly, the antibody response to the mimicking proteins, tax and hnRNP A1, has fulfilled a critical definition of molecular mimicry, that cross-reactivity between two proteins is not random but must include a biologically important region of the proteins. Our data indicate that the antibody response to the mimicking sequence of tax includes its immunodominant epitope in humans. The epitope recognized on hnRNP A1 is M9, a sequence critical to transport of the protein in and out of the nucleus, which in turn, is required for normal cell function. In addition, as shown by the intense staining of Betz cell neurons and IgG deposition of the corticospinal system in HAM/TSP autopsy specimens, immunoreactivity is specific for neurons and axons selectively damaged in HAM/TSP. Finally, cross-reactive antibodies inhibited CNS neuronal firing, indicating they are not "bystanders" but are biologically active and potentially pathogenic (Jernigan et al. 2003; Kalume et al. 2004; Levin et al. 1998, 2002a, 2002b).

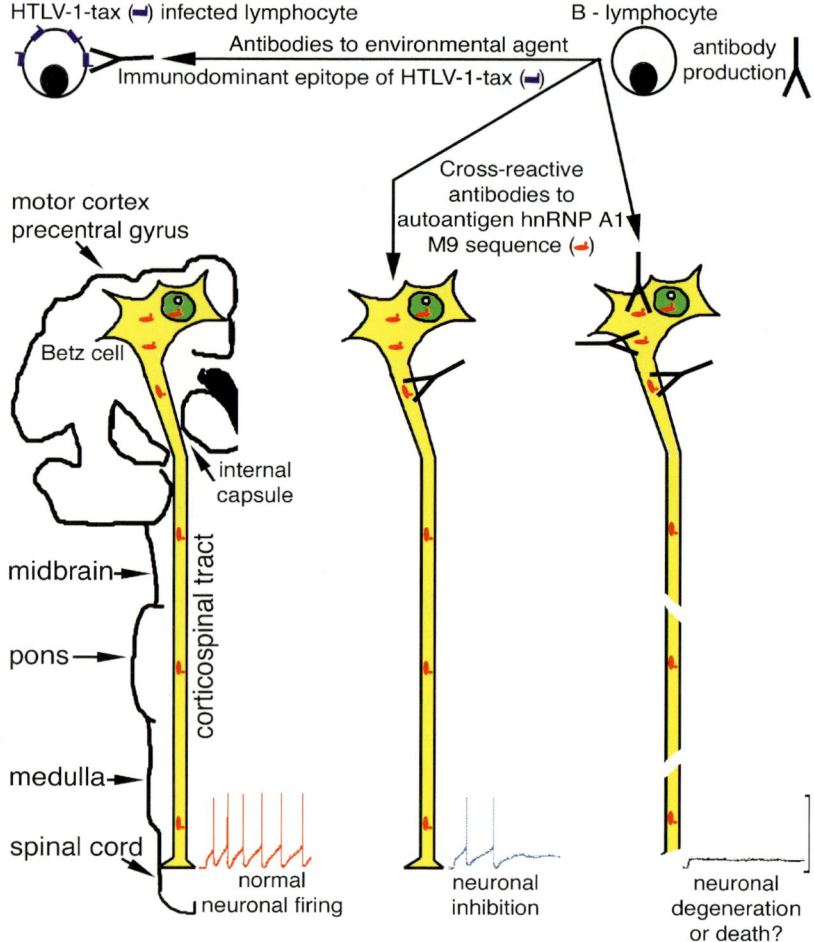

Fig. 1 The contribution of molecular mimicry between HTLV-1 and hnRNP A1 in the pathogenesis of HAM/TSP. The *left side* of the figure shows a schematic cross section of human brain that includes the pre-central gyrus. This area of motor cortex contains Betz cells whose axons make up the corticospinal tract. The corticospinal tract is shown as it courses through the internal capsule, midbrain, pons, medulla, and spinal cord. The tracing at the *bottom* of the figure shows the firing rate of motor neurons. Infection with HTLV-1 causes an antibody response to HTLV-1-tax (*top*). In this model, tax-specific antibodies immunodominant for its C terminus, cross-react with the M9 sequence of hnRNP A1 expressed by CNS neurons, particularly of corticospinal origin. This immune reaction results in inhibition of neuronal firing and potentially neurodegeneration and death

These data indicate that molecular mimicry contributes to the pathogenesis of HAM/TSP. Certainly, other immune mechanisms are also involved (Bangham 2000, 2003; Barmak et al. 2003; Jacobson 2002; Levin and Jacobson 1997; Nagai and Osame 2003; Osame 2002). Importantly, we think these data will provide valuable insights as to the cause of MS. There are important parallels between the two diseases. Clinically, some forms of MS, such as primary progressive MS, closely resemble HAM/TSP (Khan et al. 2001; Levin and Jacobson 1997). Pathologically, both diseases are associated with an activated immune response with infiltrating lymphocytes and macrophages within the CNS in areas of demyelination and axonal dystrophy (Levin and Jacobson 1997; Martin and McFarland 1995; Wu et al. 1993; Yoshioka et al. 1993). Both diseases have HLA associations and are more common in women (Jeffery et al. 1999; Martin and McFarland 1995). Interestingly, recent data suggest that infection with human herpes virus-6 (HHV-6), *Chlamydia pneumoniae,* and Epstein–Barr Virus (EBV) may contribute to the pathogenesis of MS (Lang et al. 2002; Soldan et al. 1997; Sriram et al. 1999). Thus, similar to the epidemiology of HAM/TSP, large numbers of people may be exposed to one of these common environmental agents, compared to small numbers afflicted with the disease. Remarkably, myelin basic protein, the single most studied autoantigen in MS, is transported in the oligodendrocyte by hnRNP A2, a ribonucleoprotein with significant homology to hnRNP A1 (Munro et al. 1999). Future studies may show that immunoreactivity to hnRNPs are significant contributors to the pathogenesis of autoimmune diseases of the CNS.

References

Albert LJ, Inman RD (1999) Molecular mimicry and autoimmunity. N Engl J Med 341:2068–2074
Bangham CR (2000) The immune response to HTLV-I. Curr Opin Immunol 12:397–402
Bangham CR (2003) Human T-lymphotropic virus type 1 (HTLV-1): persistence and immune control. Int J Hematol 78:297–303
Barmak K, Harhaj E, Grant C, Alefantis T, Wigdahl B (2003) Human T cell leukemia virus type I-induced disease: pathways to cancer and neurodegeneration. Virology 308:1–12
Edlich RF, Arnette JA, Williams FM (2000) Global epidemic of human T-cell lymphotropic virus type-I (HTLV-I). J Emerg Med 18:109–119
Elovaara I, Koenig S, Brewah AY, Woods RM, Lehky T, Jacobson S (1993) High human T cell lymphotropic virus type 1 (HTLV-1)-specific precursor cytotoxic T lymphocyte frequencies in patients with HTLV-1-associated neurological disease. J Exp Med 177:1567–1573
Gessain A, Vernant J, Maurs L, Barin F, Gout O, Calender A, The GD (1985) Antibodies to human T-lymphotropic virus type-I in patients with tropical spastic paraparesis. Lancet 2:407–210

Giraudon P, Szymocha R, Buart S, Bernard A, Cartier L, Belin M, Akaoka H (2000) T lymphocytes activated by persistent viral infection differentially modify the expression of metalloproteinases and their endogenous inhibitors, TIMPs, in human astrocytes: relevance to HTLV-I-induced neurological disease. J Immunol 164:2718–2727

Goon PK, Hanon E, Igakura T, Tanaka Y, Weber JN, Taylor GP, Bangham CR (2002) High frequencies of Th1-type CD4(+) T cells specific to HTLV-1 Env and Tax proteins in patients with HTLV-1-associated myelopathy/tropical spastic paraparesis. Blood 99:3335–3341

Gran B, Hemmer B, Vergelli M, McFarland H, Martin R (1999) Molecular mimicry and multiple sclerosis: degenerate T-cell recognition and the induction of autoimmunity. Ann Neurol 45:559–567

Hollsberg P, Hafler D (1993) Seminars in medicine of the Beth Israel Hospital, Boston. Pathogenesis of diseases induced by human lymphotropic virus type I infection. N Engl J Med 328:1173–1182

Izumo S, Umehara F, Osame M (2000) HTLV-I-associated myelopathy. Neuropathology [20 Suppl]:S65–68

Jacobson S (2002) Immunopathogenesis of human T cell lymphotropic virus type I-associated neurologic disease. J Infect Dis 186 [Suppl 2]:S187–192

Jacobson S, Shida H, McFarlin DE, Fauci AS, Koenig S (1990) Circulating CD8+ cytotoxic T lymphocytes specific for HTLV-I pX in patients with HTLV-I associated neurological disease. Nature 348:245–248

Jeffery KJ, Usuku K, Hall SE, Matsumoto W, Taylor GP, Procter J, Bunce M, Ogg GS, Welsh KI, Weber JN, Lloyd AL, Nowak MA, Nagai M, Kodama D, Izumo S, Osame M, Bangham CR (1999) HLA alleles determine human T-lymphotropic virus-I (HTLV-I) proviral load and the risk of HTLV-I-associated myelopathy. Proc Natl Acad Sci U S A 96:3848–5383

Jernigan M, Morcos Y, Lee SM, Dohan FC Jr, Raine C, Levin MC (2003) IgG in brain correlates with clinicopathological damage in HTLV-1 associated neurologic disease. Neurology 60:1320–1327

Kalume F, Lee SM, Morcos Y, Callaway JC, Levin MC (2004) Molecular mimicry: cross-reactive antibodies from patients with immune-mediated neurologic disease inhibit neuronal firing. J Neurosci Res 77:82–89

Khan RB, Bertorini TE, Levin MC (2001) HTLV-1 and its neurological complications. Neurologist 7:271–8

Krecic AM, Swanson MS (1999) hnRNP complexes: composition, structure, and function. Curr Opin Cell Biol 11:363–371

Lal R (1996) J Acq Imm Def Syn Human Retro 13:S170–S178

Lal RB, Giam C.-Z, Coligan, JE, Rudolph DL (1994) J Infect Dis 169:496–503

Lang H, Jacobsen H, Ikemizu S, Andersson C, Harlos K, Madsen L, Hjorth P, Sondergaard L, Svejgaard A, Wucherpfennig K, Stuart D, Bell J, Jones E, Fugger L (2002) A functional and structural basis for TCR cross-reactivity in multiple sclerosis. Nat Immunol 3:940–3

Levin M, Krichavsky M, Berk J, Foley S, Rosenfeld M, Dalmau J, Chen G, Posner J, Jacobson S (1998) Neuronal molecular mimicry in immune-mediated neurologic disease. Ann Neurol 44:87–98

Levin M, Lehky T, Flerlage N, Katz D, Kingma D, Jaffe E, Heiss J, Patronas N, McFarland H, Jacobson S (1997) New Engl J Med 336:839–845

Levin MC, Jacobson S (1997) HTLV-I associated myelopathy/tropical spastic paraparesis (HAM/TSP): a chronic progressive neurologic disease associated with immunologically mediated damage to the central nervous system.J Neurovirol 3:126–140

Levin MC, Lee SM, Kalume F, Morcos Y, Dohan FC Jr, Hasty KA, Callaway JC, Zunt J, Desiderio D, Stuart JM (2002a) Autoimmunity due to molecular mimicry as a cause of neurological disease. Nat Med 8:509–513

Levin MC, Lee SM, Morcos Y, Brady J, Stuart J (2002b) Cross-reactivity between immunodominant human T lymphotropic virus type I tax and neurons: implications for molecular mimicry. J Infect Dis 186:1514–1517

Martin R, McFarland H (1995) Immunological aspects of experimental allergic encephalomyelitis and multiple sclerosis. Crit Rev Clin Lab Sci 32:121–182

McFarlin D, Blattner WB (1991) Annu Rev Med 42:97–105

Moore G, Traugott U, Scheinberg L, Raine C (1989) Tropical spastic paraparesis: a model of virus-induced, cytotoxic T-cell-mediated demyelination? Ann Neurol 26:523–530

Muller S, Boire G, Ossondo M, Ricchiuti V, Smadja D, Vernant J.-C, Ozden S (1995) IgG autoantibody response in HTLV-I-infected patients. Clin Immunol Immunopathol 77:282–290

Munro TP, Magee RJ, Kidd GJ, Carson JH, Barbarese E, Smith LM, Smith R (1999) Mutational analysis of a heterogeneous nuclear ribonucleoprotein A2 response element for RNA trafficking. J Biol Chem 274:34389–34395

Nagai M, Osame M (2003) Human T-cell lymphotropic virus type I and neurological diseases. J Neurovirol 9:228–235

Nagai M, Usuku K, Matsumoto W, Kodama D, Takenouchi N, Moritoyo T, Hashiguchi S, Ichinose M, Bangham CR, Izumo S, Osame M (1998) Analysis of HTLV-I proviral load in 202 HAM/TSP patients and 243 asymptomatic HTLV-I carriers: high proviral load strongly predisposes to HAM/TSP. J Neurovirol 4:586–593

Nakagawa M, Izumo S, Ijichi S, Kubota H, Arimura K, Kawabata M, Osame M (1995) HTLV-I-associated myelopathy: analysis of 213 patients based on clinical features and laboratory findings. J Neurovirol 1:50–61

Nakielny S, Dreyfuss G (1997) Curr Opin Cell Biol 9:420–429

Niewiesk S, Daenke S, Parker CE, Taylor G, Weber J, Nightingale S, Bangham CR (1994) The transactivator gene of human T-cell leukemia virus type I is more variable within and between healthy carriers than patients with tropical spastic paraparesis. J Virol 68:6778–81

Noraz N, Benichou S, Madaule P, Tiollais P, Vernant J, Degranges C (1993) Expression of HTLV-I Env and Tax recombinant peptides in yeast: identification of immunogenic domains. Virology 193:80–88

Oldstone M (1998) Molecular mimicry and immune-mediated diseases. FASEB J 12:1255–1265

Osame M (2002) Pathological mechanisms of human T-cell lymphotropic virus type I-associated myelopathy (HAM/TSP). J Neurovirol 8:359–364

Osame M, Matsumoto M, Usuku K, Izumo S, Ijichi N, Amitani H, Tara M, Igata A (1987) Chronic progressive myelopathy associated with elevated antibodies to human T-lymphotropic virus type I and adult T-cell leukemialike cells. Ann Neurol 21:117–122

Osame M, Usuku K, Izumo S, Ijichi N, Amitani H, Igata A, Matsumoto M, Tara M (1986) HTLV-I associated myelopathy, a new clinical entity. Lancet 1:1031–1032

Poeisz B, Ruscetti F, Gazdar A, Bunn P, Minna J, Gallo R (1980) Detection and isolation of type C retrovirus particles from fresh and cultured lymphocytes of a patient with cutaneous T-cell lymphoma. Proc Natl Acad Sci U S A 77:7415–7419

Romero I, Prevost M, Perret E, Adamson P, Greenwood J, Couraud P, Ozden S (2000) Interactions between brain endothelial cells and human T-cell leukemia virus type 1-infected lymphocytes: mechanisms of viral entry into the central nervous system. J Virol 74:6021–6030

Rudolph DL, Coligan JE, Lal RB (1994) Detection of antibodies to trans-activator protein (p40taxI) of human T-cell lymphotropic virus type I by a synthetic peptide-based assay. Clin Diagn Lab Immunol March:176–181

Saito M, Nakagawa M, Kaseda S, Matsuzaki T, Jonosono M, Eiraku N, Kubota R, Takenouchi N, Nagai M, Furukawa Y, Usuku K, Izumo S, Osame M (2004) Decreased human T lymphotropic virus type I (HTLV-I) provirus load and alteration in T cell phenotype after interferon-alpha therapy for HTLV-I-associated myelopathy/tropical spastic paraparesis. J Infect Dis 189:29–40

Shyu A-B, Wilkinson MF (2000) The double lives of shuttling mRNA binding proteins. Cell 102:135–138

Soldan S, Berti R, Salem N, Secchiero P, Flamand L, Calabresi P, Brennan M, Maloni H, McFarland H, Lin H.-C, Patnaik M, Jacobson S (1997) Association of human herpes virus 6 (HHV-6) with multiple sclerosis: increased IgM response to HHV-6 early antigen and detection of serum HHV-6 DNA. Nat Med 3:1394–1397

Sriram S, Stratton C, Yao S, Tharp A, Ding L, Bannan J, Mitchell W (1999) Chlamydia pneumoniae infection of the central nervous system in multiple sclerosis. Ann Neurol 46:6–14

Umehara F, Itoh K, Michizono K, Abe M, Izumo S, Osame M (2002) Involvement of Fas/Fas ligand system in the spinal cords of HTLV-I-associated myelopathy. Acta Neuropathol (Berl) 103:384–90

Umehara F, Okada Y, Fujimoto N, Abe M, Izumo S, Osame M (1998) Expression of matrix metalloproteinases and tissue inhibitors of metalloproteinases in HTLV-I-associated myelopathy. J Neuropathol Exp Neurol 57:839–49

Wu E, Dickson D, Jacobson S, Raine C (1993) Neuroaxonal dystrophy in HTLV-1-associated myelopathy/tropical spastic paraparesis: neuropathologic and neuroimmunologic correlations. Acta Neuropathol 86:224–235

Wucherpfennig KW (2002) Nat Med 8:455–457

Yoshida M, Osame M, Usuku K, Matsumoto M, Igata A (1987) Viruses detected in HTLV-I-associated myelopathy and adult T-cell leukaemia are identical on DNA blotting. Lancet 1:1085–1086

Yoshioka A, Hirose G, Ueda Y, Nishimura Y, Sakai K (1993) Neuropathological studies of the spinal cord in early stage HTLV-I-associated myelopathy (HAM). J Neurol Neurosurg Psych 56:1004–7

Molecular Mimicry: Anti-DNA Antibodies Bind Microbial and Nonnucleic Acid Self-Antigens

J. S. Rice[1] · C. Kowal[2] · B. T. Volpe[3] · L. A. DeGiorgio[3] · B. Diamond[4] (✉)

[1]Integrated Department of Immunology, National Jewish Medical Research Center, University of Colorado Health Sciences Center, 1400 Jackson St, K806, Denver, CO 80206, USA

[2]Department of Medicine, Columbia University Medical Center, 1130 St. Nicholas Avenue, Audobon III Bldg. 9th Fl. Rm 916, New York, NY 10032, USA

[3]Department of Neurology and Neuroscience, The Burke Medical Research Institute, Weill Medical College of Cornell University, 785 Mamaroneck Avenue, White Plains, New York, NY 10605, USA

[4]Department of Medicine, Division of Rheumatology, Columbia University Medical Center, 630 West 168th Street PH8E Suite 101, New York, NY 10032, USA
bd2137@Columbia.edu

1	Introduction	138
2	Induction of Anti-DNA Antibodies	138
3	Cross-Reactivity Among Self-Antigens	140
4	Anti-DNA Antibody Reactivity with NMDA Receptors	140
5	Autoreactivity in the CNS	141
5.1	Neurological Disease in SLE	142
6	Lupus Antibodies Cause Neuronal Damage In Vivo	143
7	Epinephrine Opens the BBB	146
8	Conclusion	146
References		147

Abstract Although cells of the innate immune response have a variety of pattern recognition receptors that are triggered by blood classes of markers, a critical feature of the adaptive immune response is antigenic specificity. Yet it is becoming increasingly clear that the specificity of lymphocyte receptors admits of some laxity. Cross-reactivity may, in fact, be necessary for lymphocyte survival as antigen receptor signaling maintains cellular viability in the absence of antigen activation. Studies of molecular mimicry have revealed many instances in which antibodies to microbial antigens bind also to self-antigens; in some cases, this cross-reactivity has pathogenic potential. In this chapter, we describe cross-reactivity between two self-antigens, DNA and NMDA receptors, and how antibodies with specificity for DNA in patients with splenic lupus may cause central nervous system damage by virtue of binding also to neuronal receptors. This example serves as a reminder that cross-reactivity may exist among self-antigens as well as between foreign and self-antigens.

1
Introduction

Systemic lupus erythematosus (SLE) is a rheumatic disorder and, like many autoimmune diseases, primarily affects women. Complications involving the central nervous system (CNS) are frequently reported, with the percentage of patients displaying CNS symptoms varying from 15% to 85%, depending on the instrument used for clinical assessment as well as the patient cohort. Symptoms include headache, migraines, seizures, chorea, as well as cognitive decline and psychiatric manifestations such as anxiety, mood disorder, and psychosis (Kozora et al. 1996). Whether the CNS disorders observed in SLE are a result of the direct impact of the immune system on neuronal function, a consequence of vascular disease or hypertension, or a result of pharmacological interventions has been unclear. We have recently shown that anti-DNA antibodies, the signature autospecificity in SLE and known to cause renal disease, can cross-react with NMDA receptors expressed on neurons (DeGiorgio et al. 2001). This binding causes neuronal death, leading to altered behavior and impaired cognition (Kowal et al. 2004). This observation represents an example of molecular mimicry, with autoantibodies recognizing multiple self-antigens, and perhaps mediating damage through multiple mechanisms.

2
Induction of Anti-DNA Antibodies

Normal immune system function requires a balancing of the ability to respond to foreign challenge with the necessity of remaining nonresponsive to self molecules. Achieving immunity and maintaining tolerance involve multiple mechanisms, including negative selection regulatory networks and immune privilege. SLE is an autoimmune disease characterized by anti-nuclear antibodies, especially antibodies to double-stranded (ds) DNA. There has long been a question regarding the trigger for the production of these antibodies. Recent studies from murine models of SLE have clearly shown that on a permissive genetic background the failure to clear apoptotic cells can lead to the production of anti-DNA antibodies (Licht et al. 2004; Potter et al. 2003). There is scant evidence, however, that many patients fail to clear apoptotic debris; thus it remains unclear whether this is a major trigger of anti-DNA antibody production in SLE. One alterative hypothesis has always been that anti-DNA antibodies arise by molecular mimicry.

We have long been interested in identifying microbial antigens that might induce production of anti-DNA antibodies in a host with poor regulation of autoreactivity. Some time ago we showed that an antibody to phosphorylcholine (PC), a dominant epitope on pneumococcal cell wall polysaccharide, could acquire a single amino acid substitution and gain specificity for dsDNA (Diamond and Scharff 1984). We subsequently showed that in a non-lupus-prone mouse strain, approximately 40% of the B cells responding to immunization with PC coupled to a protein carrier cross-react with dsDNA. These B cells mature in germinal center reactions but are eliminated before entering the memory B cell compartment. On the basis of this finding, we postulated that lupus-prone individuals may have poor negative selection of the B cell repertoire or inadequate immune regulation. Under abnormal conditions, such as may exist in SLE, some of the B cells that acquire autospecificity after antigen activation may mature into plasma cells and memory B cells and lead to elevated serum anti-DNA reactivity. We subsequently demonstrated that approximately half of the anti-pneumococcal antibodies present in a combinatorial library made from spleen cells of a lupus patient vaccinated with pneumococcal polysaccharide before therapeutic splenectomy cross-react with DNA. We have also shown that serum anti-DNA antibodies cross-react with pneumococcal polysaccharide and that anti-DNA antibodies are somatically mutated. These observations make it plausible that poor regulation of somatically mutating B cells that have been activated by microbial antigen can lead to autoantibody production. Others have shown that anti-DNA antibodies can cross-react with other microbial antigens. Recently, there have been studies suggesting that EBV infection may predispose to SLE, and anti-viral antibodies may cross-react with nuclear antigens (Stein et al. 2002). In composite, these studies suggest that many microbial antigens may elicit anti-DNA antibodies in a susceptible host. It is therefore appealing to speculate that a B cell repertoire established with an inadequate threshold for the elimination of autoreactivity leads to autoreactivity in the response to microbial antigen and fails to focus the anti-microbial response on protective antigenic epitopes. Thus, diminished protective immunity may accompany autoimmunity.

3
Cross-Reactivity Among Self-Antigens

Anti-DNA antibodies not only cross-react with microbial antigens; there is also an extensive literature on self-antigens bound by anti-DNA antibodies. These studies have focused on renal antigens that might be bound in glomeruli by anti-DNA antibodies, leading to an inflammatory response and to lupus nephritis. Among the antigens bound by anti-DNA antibodies and present in glomeruli are heparan sulfate, laminin, and alpha actinin (Deocharan et al. 2002; Faaber et al. 1986; Sabbaga et al. 1989). It has not been conclusively shown that anti-DNA antibodies with one or more of these cross-reactivities deposit in glomeruli by virtue of the binding to extracellular matrix components, but it has been demonstrated that antibodies will bind glomeruli even after the glomeruli have been treated with DNase (Venkatesh and Diamond 2004). Many of these cross-reactive antigens will also trigger production of anti-DNA antibodies when administered to mice in a strong adjuvant. There are currently no compelling data, however, to suggest that these nonnucleic acid self-antigens are presented in an immunogenic fashion in SLE and constitute the trigger for anti-DNA antibody production. In particular, T cell reactivity to these antigens has not been demonstrated Rather, they represent target antigens for tissue damage.

4
Anti-DNA Antibody Reactivity with NMDA Receptors

Motivated by studies showing that protein antigens can be the target tissue antigen bound by anti-DNA antibodies, and looking to determine whether some protein antigens might elicit anti-DNA antibodies in SLE, we elected to screen a phage peptide display library with a murine anti-DNA antibody, R4A, capable of binding to glomeruli. The screening revealed that the consensus sequence Asp/Glu-Trp-Asp/Glu-Tyr-Ser/Gly (DWEYS) was bound by this antibody (Gaynor et al. 1997). Immunization with this sequence on a carrier protein induces an antibody response to both peptide and dsDNA in BALB/c mice, a strain that is not spontaneously prone to develop autoantibodies. The induced antibodies deposit in glomeruli and result in proteinuria (Putterman and Diamond 1998). The consensus sequence of this peptide is present in pneumococcal choline kinase. Immunization of BALB/c mice with choline kinase leads to the development of high titers of anti-DNA antibodies, thereby identifying yet another microbial antigen capable of eliciting anti-DNA antibodies (Kowal and Diamond 2004; unpublished data).

This peptide motif is also present in the extracellular, ligand-binding domain of both mouse and human N-methyl-D-aspartate (NMDA) receptor subunits NR2a and NR2b. These receptors are widely expressed by neurons in the forebrain, and they bind the neurotransmitter glutamate (Kosinski et al. 1998, Kuppenbender et al. 2000; Scherzer et al. 1998; Standaert et al. 1994). Glutamate receptors are involved in memory and learning (Morris et al. 1986), they display altered expression in psychosis, and overstimulation of these receptors can cause neuronal apoptosis (Akbarian et al. 1996; Choi and Rothman 1990; Mattson et al. 2000). In light of the similarity between NMDA receptor function and the observed cognitive deficits observed in lupus patients, combined with the presence of the consensus motif in the receptor, we sought evidence for a mechanism mediated by cross-reactive anti-DNA antibodies. Western blot analysis confirmed that anti-dsDNA antibodies bound NR2-containing receptors (DeGiorgio et al. 2001).

5
Autoreactivity in the CNS

Autoimmunity within the CNS has been studied primarily in multiple sclerosis (MS) and in rodent models of MS, which are characterized by an inflammatory infiltrate in the brain and subsequent demyelination. Cognitive and motor defects, as well as certain personality disorders, are present in MS and in other autoimmune disorders, including SLE, and postinfectious autoimmunity (Paul et al. 1998; Ring et al. 1998), but the link between the neurological syndromes and the autoreactivity that can be detected in serum or peripheral blood cells is unclear. Most surprisingly, it has been proposed by some that the immune system contributes to the development and pathogenesis of neuropsychiatric disorders (Fessel 1962); however, the mechanisms of immune modulation of neuronal function have largely remained unclear.

Brain-reactive autoantibodies (BRAAs) have been reported in patients with a range of neurological and psychiatric disorders, including SLE, antiphospholipid syndrome, myasthenia gravis, Lambert-Eaton syndrome, Sydenham chorea, Guillain-Barré syndrome, schizophrenia, Sjögren's syndrome, chronic fatigue syndrome, autism, motor neuron disease, neuromyotonia, paraneoplastic cerebellar degeneration, Rasmussen encephalitis, as well as HIV-related dementia (Aarli 2000; Ang et al. 2004; Cavill et al. 2004; Kim and Neher 1988; Leveque et al. 1992; Rutter et al. 1987; Rutter and Schopler 1987; Sastre-Garriga and Montalban 2003; Schutzer et al. 2003; Sinha et al. 1991; Tanaka et al. 2003; Vojdani et al. 2002; Waterhouse et al. 1991). Connections are also being sought between autoimmunity and disorders such as fibromyalgia, Gulf War syndrome, sudden infant death syndrome, and chronic Lyme disease of the CNS (Martin et al. 2001; Staines 2004a, 2004b, 2004c).

It continues to be debated whether BRAAs are an effector of neuronal damage or a marker of disease that arises subsequent to alterations in brain antigenicity, vasculature, or function. In some situations, there is evidence that infection triggers the generation of autoantibodies through the mechanism of molecular mimicry. In others, it has been argued that autoreactivity occurs secondary to brain injury and the ensuing autoimmune response reflects a novel exposure of mature lymphocytes to brain antigens. Although neurological syndromes often arise during autoimmune diseases, the nature of their link to the autoreactivity itself has, remained unclear. Thrombotic events and vascular alterations often accompany autoimmunity (Trivedi and Bussel 2003). These can predispose to the presentation of brain antigen by activated dendritic cells. Moreover, autoimmunity may cause inflammation and compromise the blood-brain barrier (BBB), which may result in neurological side-effects that are not directly related to a new loss of self-tolerance, but rather the exposure of brain tissue to antibodies in the systemic circulation. Finally, neuropathology often develops slowly and may not be identified until after the instigating pathogen has been cleared. Thus, identifying the primary infection may be challenging, and proof linking an infection to neuropsychiatric symptoms may be elusive.

5.1
Neurological Disease in SLE

An intriguing feature of many of the neurological symptoms that develop in lupus patients is the discordance between symptoms and disease flares. We hypothesize that this is a reflection of the immune-privileged nature of the CNS. Because the CNS is protected from immune assault by the presence of the BBB, two insults may be required for neurological disease to develop: One insult results in the development of an antineuronal response, and a second insult breaks the BBB and allows autoantibodies to reach their target antigens. Breakdown of the BBB may be a feature of disease activity, such as vasculitis or other vascular involvement, or may be due to an event independent of disease activity such as infection or stress (Abdel-Rahman et al. 2002; Esposito et al. 2002; Friedman et al. 1996; Xaio et al. 2001). Thus tissue damage in the CNS may occur with or without disease activity so long as autoantibodies are present in the systemic circulation.

The actual role of autoantibodies in neuropsychiatric lupus remains controversial. Studies of MRL/lpr mice, which spontaneously develop a lupuslike disease, have revealed neurological defects including diminished learning and memory capacity (Szechtman et al. 1997). These defects have been linked to the development of autoimmune disease, rather than to an innate genetic defect in the strain (Sakic et al. 1992; Sherman et al. 1990). Neurodegeneration present in older MRL/lpr mice occurs in conjunction with the infiltration of activated T cells into the CNS and the presence of neurotoxic autoantibodies in the cerebrospinal fluid, and correlates with behavioral changes (Ballok et al. 2004b). Mice are at least partially protected from the development of neurodegeneration by immunosuppressive therapy (Sakic et al. 2000). A link between autoantibodies, hippocampal dysfunction, and behavior abnormalities has recently been noted, and is associated with the presence of apoptotic neurons in the CA3 region of the hippocampus (Ballok et al. 2004a). This finding was also noted in a post-mortem analysis of a patient who died of SLE. Although BRAAs were identified in the serum of affected mice, a causal relationship between the autoantibodies and the onset of neurological disease was not demonstrated. Specifically, it is not known whether BRAAs are the mechanism for neuronal death, or a marker for neuronal injury mediated by another mechanism. Moreover, cellular infiltrates have been observed in the brains of MRL/lpr mice and could represent a cell-mediated mechanism for neuronal death (Kier 1990). This stands in contrast to the antibody-mediated model we have explored.

6
Lupus Antibodies Cause Neuronal Damage In Vivo

Once we determined that the R4A anti-DNA antibody bound a consensus sequence present in NR2-containing receptors and bound to NMDA receptors, we demonstrated that purified R4A antibody injected into the hippocampus of non-autoimmune mice resulted in neuronal loss (DeGiorgio et al. 2001). Fab'2 fragments of the antibody also mediated neuronal death, indicating a mechanism that is independent of complement activation or the activation of Fc-receptor bearing cells in the brain. Serum antibodies from lupus patients purified on a peptide affinity column bound NR2 and dsDNA, confirming the cross-reactivity we had initially observed. These antibodies also induced neuronal apoptosis when injected into the hippocampus. Furthermore, when the NMDA receptor antagonist MK801 was given systemically to mice, it protected against neuronal death induced by direct injection of antibody into the hippocampus. Several important observations were therefore made. First, neuronal apoptosis occurred in the absence of any cellular infiltrate. Second, cell death was not dependent on complement or cell-mediated pathways, as anti-NR2 Fab'2 fragments were also able to induce death. Finally, mice pretreated with MK-801, an NR2 blocker, were protected from antibody-mediated neuronal damage, strongly indicating that R4A binding induced cellular signaling. Thus the mechanism of neuronal death was determined to be dependent on antibody-mediated neuronal activation. The antibody therefore appeared to function as a receptor agonist, and to mediate apoptosis through excitotoxicity.

In nonspontaneously autoimmune BALB/c mice immunized with the DNA peptide mimetope DWEYS coupled to a multi-antigenic poly-lysine backbone (MAP), high serum titers of anti-peptide antibodies arise (Gaynor et al. 1997). These autoantibodies have pathogenic potential as they deposit in renal glomeruli and cause proteinuria and a mild inflammatory reaction (Gaynor et al. 1997; Putterman and Diamond 1998). An examination of the brains of these mice revealed no neuronal damage, no infiltration of inflammatory cells, and no immunoglobulin deposition in the cortex or hippocampus (Kowal et al. 2004). These data confirmed the importance of the BBB; reactivity of serum with brain antigens is insufficient for neuropathology to develop a breach in the BBB.

The BBB constitutes a significant protective mechanism to shield the CNS from potentially pathogenic infectious or inflammatory agents. Presumably, although tissue destruction accompanying an immune response may be tolerated to varying degrees in other tissues, the loss of even small numbers of neuronal cells may be devastating. Moreover, inflammation can have significant pathogenic effects on the CNS, as the brain is anatomically constrained by the skull. Thus the movement of cells and small molecules into and out of the CNS is actively controlled by cells making up the BBB, and most molecules that cross the membrane do so by means of active transport (Pardridge 1998). Multiple mechanisms are known to open the BBB that are of particular importance in SLE. Both infection and stress may result in opening of the BBB (Oztas et al. 2004) and expose autoreactive antibodies to tissues where they may influence neurological function. Studies have shown that epinephrine can induce opening of the BBB (Banks 2001). Bacterial antigens, such as lipopolysaccharide (LPS), can also increase BBB permeability (Xaio et al. 2001), and it has been demonstrated in vivo that some bacterial infections, like streptococcus, can induce opening of the BBB (Paul et al. 1998; Ring et al. 1998). This is of particular interest in light of recent observations that the consensus sequence bound by the antibody R4A, and appearing in the glutamate receptor, also appears in the enzyme choline kinase of *Streptococcus pneumonia* and that immunization with choline kinase induces anti-DNA anti-peptide antibodies (Kowal and Diamond 2004). Finally, sex hormones can modulate permeability of the BBB (Oztas 1998), possibly explaining the increased incidence of certain autoimmune neurological syndromes during pregnancy (Cervera et al. 1997).

Previous reports have indicated that when LPS opens the BBB, there is no resulting brain pathology (Xaio et al. 2001). Therefore we administered LPS by intraperitoneal injection to mice were immunized with the dsDNA mimetope DWEYS. At 1 week after LPS administration, intense immunoglobulin deposition was observed in the hippocampal neurons (Kowal et al. 2004). Examination of the brains of these mice revealed extensive hippocampal neuronal loss in the absence of inflammation, especially of pyramidal neurons in the CA1 region of the hippocampus. To further confirm the regional specificity of the damage to these mice, magnetic resonance spectroscopy was used to probe brain metabolism. Measurement of the brain metabolite N-acetyl aspartate (NAA) and of the ratio of NAA to creatine (Cr) permits the identification of areas of neuronal loss (Hetherington et al. 1995; Hugg et al. 1993). Mice immunized with the dsDNA mimetope developed anti-NR2 antibodies and displayed decreased NAA-to-Cr ratios in the hippocampus consistent with neuronal loss when the BBB was compromised by LPS. This effect was not seen after LPS treatment in mice immunized with the carrier alone. Moreover, behavior studies in these immunized mice treated with LPS revealed cognitive deficits. Specifically, mice performed poorly in challenges that tested hippocampal function; these defects were especially evident in memory trials (Kowal et al. 2004). The cognitive dysfunction found in these mice parallels similar patterns of cognitive performance found in lupus patients (Brey et al. 2002; Denburg and Denburg 1999).

Confirmation that neuronal damage occurred as a consequence of signaling through NMDA receptors was obtained with the inhibitor memantine. Memantine is a selective inhibitor of NR2A- and NR2B-containing receptors (Avenet et al. 1997; Danysz and Parsons 2003). Nonautoimmune BALB/c mice were immunized with DWEYS, resulting in anti-peptide, anti-dsDNA, and anti-NR2 antibodies. As previously mentioned, treatment with LPS resulted in an opening of the BBB and subsequent neuropathology. However, administration of the NR2-inhibitor memantine before LPS protected mice from neuronal apoptosis, despite significant anti-NR2 antibody titers (Kowal et al. 2004). No hippocampal injury was observed, and no Fluoro Jade staining or activated caspase was detected. This confirmed that autoantibody-mediated cell signaling by NR2-containing receptors was responsible for the observed neuronal damage.

7
Epinephrine Opens the BBB

In addition to LPS, which may be present during bacterial infection, studies also show that stress can induce BBB opening. Epinephrine has been shown to increase BBB permeability (Oztas et al. 2004) and was explored in this model. We administered epinephrine systemically to DWEYS peptide-immunized mice. Of interest, the hippocampus is spared after epinephrine administration but there is apoptosis of cells in the amygdala. These mice perform normally in tests of memory function but fail to respond to a fear-conditioning paradigm. The histology in the amygdala, as in the hippocampus, reveals an absence of inflammatory cell activation. Thus we have evidence that antibodies can mediate both cognitive and behavioral changes by functioning as receptor agonists.

8
Conclusion

A significant obstacle to the interpretation of autoimmune-mediated neurological syndromes is that disease flares do not correlate well with neurological status. This might reflect the fact that neurological symptoms may not be detected until the putative instigating infection has been cleared. The model we propose for autoimmune neuropathologies, specifically neuropsychiatric lupus, is a two-part model. Initially, autoimmunity arises that contains reactivity to brain antigens. This autoimmunity may be a product of cross-reactivity from an infection or of cross-reactivity to other self-antigens that are triggers for autoantibody production. However, as we have reported, the presence of BRAAs in the serum alone is not sufficient for the development of neurological disease (Kowal et al. 2004). There must be an abrogation of the BBB and antibody access to brain tissue.

Recent studies have provided strong evidence that anti-neuronal antibodies can arise in the course of immune reactions to foreign antigens (Kalume et al. 2004; Kirvan et al. 2003; Kowal et al. 2004). Not only are these antibodies capable of binding to neuronal surface antigens, but they have been shown to be capable of modulating neuronal function as both stimulatory and inhibitory molecules. These mechanisms have parallels in pharmaceutical agents that are known to mediate their cognitive effects by apparently similar mechanisms (Heresco-Levy and Javitt 1998; Marino and Conn 2002). Moreover, it is highly significant that studies have identified the targets of several BRAAs to be targets of psychiatric pharmaceuticals.

The model of neurological disease as a result of an immune-mediated, noninflammatory neuronal loss suggests a new mechanism of disease development. Immune- and autoantibody-mediated neuropathologies are implicated or suspected in a number of psychiatric diseases, and it seems likely that the contribution of the immune system in these disorders has only begun to be appreciated. The conditions under which neuropathogenic antibodies develop require additional investigation, especially as it becomes clear that foreign antigens and possibly vaccines can elicit unanticipated cross-reactivities. Coupled with this knowledge, we must be aware of how this reactivity interacts with the nervous system, and how changes in blood-brain permeability influence disease development. These challenges will require a new synergy between the fields of neurology and immunology.

References

Aarli, JA (2000) Epilepsy and the immune system. Arch Neurol 57, 1689–92

Abdel-Rahman, A, Shetty, AK, Abou-Donia, MB (2002) Disruption of the blood-brain barrier and neuronal cell death in cingulate cortex, dentate gyrus, thalamus, and hypothalamus in a rat model of Gulf-War syndrome. Neurobiol Dis 10, 306–26

Akbarian, S, Sucher, NJ, Bradley, D, Tafazzoli, A, Trinh, D, Hetrick, WP, Potkin, SG, Sandman, CA, Bunney, WE, Jr., Jones, EG (1996) Selective alterations in gene expression for NMDA receptor subunits in prefrontal cortex of schizophrenics. J Neurosci 16, 19–30

Ang, CW, Jacobs, BC, Laman, JD (2004) The Guillain-Barre syndrome: a true case of molecular mimicry. Trends Immunol 25, 61–6

Avenet, P, Leonardon, J, Besnard, F, Graham, D, Depoortere, H, Scatton, B (1997) Antagonist properties of eliprodil and other NMDA receptor antagonists at rat NR1A/NR2A and NR1A/NR2B receptors expressed in *Xenopus* oocytes. Neurosci Lett 223, 133–6

Ballok, DA, Woulfe, J, Sur, M, Cyr, M, Sakic, B (2004a) Hippocampal damage in mouse and human forms of systemic autoimmune disease. Hippocampus 14, 649–61

Ballok, DA, Earls, AM, Krasnik, C, Hoffman, SA, Sakic, B (2004b) Autoimmune-induced damage of the midbrain dopaminergic system in lupus-prone mice. J Neuroimmunol 152, 83–97

Banks, WA (2001) Enhanced leptin transport across the blood-brain barrier by alpha 1-adrenergic agents. Brain Res 899, 209–17

Brey, RL, Holliday, SL, Saklad, AR, Navarrete, MG, Hermosillo-Romo, D, Stallworth, CL, Valdez, CR, Escalante, A, del Rincon, I, Gronseth, G, Rhine, CB, Padilla, P, McGlasson, D (2002) Neuropsychiatric syndromes in lupus: prevalence using standardized definitions. Neurology 58, 1214–20

Cavill, D, Waterman, SA, Gordon, TP (2004) Antibodies raised against the second extracellular loop of the human muscarinic M3 receptor mimic functional autoantibodies in Sjogren's syndrome. Scand J Immunol 59, 261–6

Cervera, R, Asherson, RA, Font, J, Tikly, M, Pallares, L, Chamorro, A, Ingelmo, M (1997) Chorea in the antiphospholipid syndrome. Clinical, radiologic, and immunologic characteristics of 50 patients from our clinics and the recent literature. Medicine (Baltimore) 76, 203–12

Choi, DW, Rothman, SM (1990) The role of glutamate neurotoxicity in hypoxic-ischemic neuronal death. Annu Rev Neurosci 13, 171–82

Danysz, W, Parsons, CG (2003) The NMDA receptor antagonist memantine as a symptomatological and neuroprotective treatment for Alzheimer's disease: preclinical evidence. Int J Geriatr Psychiatry 18, S23–32

DeGiorgio, LA, Konstantinov, KN, Lee, SC, Hardin, JA, Volpe, BT, Diamond, B (2001) A subset of lupus anti-DNA antibodies cross-reacts with the NR2 glutamate receptor in systemic lupus erythematosus. Nat Med 7, 1189–93

Denburg, SD, Denburg, JA (1999) Cognitive dysfunction in systemic lupus erythematosus. *In* Systemic Lupus Erythematosus (R. G. Lahita, ed.), pp. 611–629. Academic Press, San Diego

Deocharan, B, Qing, X, Lichauco, J, Putterman, C (2002) Alpha-actinin is a cross-reactive renal target for pathogenic anti-DNA antibodies. J Immunol 168, 3072–8

Diamond, B, Scharff, MD (1984) Somatic mutation of the T15 heavy chain gives rise to an antibody with autoantibody specificity. Proc Natl Acad Sci U S A 81, 5841–4

Esposito, P, Chandler, N, Kandere, K, Basu, S, Jacobson, S, Connolly, R, Tutor, D, Theoharides, TC (2002) Corticotropin-releasing hormone and brain mast cells regulate blood-brain-barrier permeability induced by acute stress. J Pharmacol Exp Ther 303, 1061–6

Faaber, P, Rijke, TP, van de Putte, LB, Capel, PJ, Berden, JH (1986) Cross-reactivity of human and murine anti-DNA antibodies with heparan sulfate. The major glycosaminoglycan in glomerular basement membranes. J Clin Invest 77, 1824–30

Fessel, WJ (1962) Autoimmunity and mental illness. A preliminary report. Arch Gen Psychiatry 6, 320–3

Friedman, A, Kaufer, D, Shemer, J, Hendler, I, Soreq, H, Tur-Kaspa, I (1996) Pyridostigmine brain penetration under stress enhances neuronal excitability and induces early immediate transcriptional response. Nat Med 2, 1382–5

Gaynor, B, Putterman, C, Valadon, P, Spatz, L, Scharff, MD, Diamond, B (1997) Peptide inhibition of glomerular deposition of an anti-DNA antibody. Proc Natl Acad Sci U S A 94, 1955–60

Heresco-Levy, U, Javitt, DC (1998) The role of N-methyl-D-aspartate (NMDA) receptor-mediated neurotransmission in the pathophysiology and therapeutics of psychiatric syndromes. Eur Neuropsychopharmacol 8, 141–52

Hetherington, H, Kuzniecky, R, Pan, J, Mason, G, Morawetz, R, Harris, C, Faught, E, Vaughan, T, Pohost, G (1995) Proton nuclear magnetic resonance spectroscopic imaging of human temporal lobe epilepsy at 4.1 T. Ann Neurol 38, 396–404

Hugg, JW, Laxer, KD, Matson, GB, Maudsley, AA, Weiner, MW (1993) Neuron loss localizes human temporal lobe epilepsy by in vivo proton magnetic resonance spectroscopic imaging. Ann Neurol 34, 788–94

Kalume, F, Lee, SM, Morcos, Y, Callaway, JC, Levin, MC (2004) Molecular mimicry: cross-reactive antibodies from patients with immune-mediated neurologic disease inhibit neuronal firing. J Neurosci Res 77, 82–9

Kier, AB (1990) Clinical neurology and brain histopathology in NZB/NZW F1 lupus mice. J Comp Pathol 102, 165–77

Kim, YI, Neher, E (1988) IgG from patients with Lambert-Eaton syndrome blocks voltage-dependent calcium channels. Science 239, 405–8

Kirvan, CA, Swedo, SE, Heuser, JS, Cunningham, MW (2003) Mimicry and autoantibody-mediated neuronal cell signaling in Sydenham chorea. Nat Med 9, 914–20

Kosinski, CM, Standaert, DG, Counihan, TJ, Scherzer, CR, Kerner, JA, Daggett, LP, Velicelebi, G, Penney, JB, Young, AB, Landwehrmeyer, GB (1998) Expression of N-methyl-D-aspartate receptor subunit mRNAs in the human brain: striatum and globus pallidus. J Comp Neurol 390, 63–74

Kowal, C, Diamond, B (2004) Unpublished observations

Kowal, C, DeGiorgio, LA, Nakaoka, T, Hetherington, H, Huerta, PT, Diamond, B, Volpe, BT (2004) Cognition and immunity; antibody impairs memory. Immunity 21, 179–88

Kozora, E, Thompson, LL, West, SG, Kotzin, BL (1996) Analysis of cognitive and psychological deficits in systemic lupus erythematosus patients without overt central nervous system disease. Arthritis Rheum 39, 2035–45

Kuppenbender, KD, Standaert, DG, Feuerstein, TJ, Penney, JB, Jr., Young, AB, Landwehrmeyer, GB (2000) Expression of NMDA receptor subunit mRNAs in neurochemically identified projection and interneurons in the human striatum. J Comp Neurol 419, 407–21

Leveque, C, Hoshino, T, David, P, Shoji-Kasai, Y, Leys, K, Omori, A, Lang, B, el Far, O, Sato, K, Martin-Moutot, N, et al (1992) The synaptic vesicle protein synaptotagmin associates with calcium channels and is a putative Lambert-Eaton myasthenic syndrome antigen. Proc Natl Acad Sci U S A 89, 3625–9

Licht, R, Dieker, JW, Jacobs, CW, Tax, WJ, Berden, JH (2004) Decreased phagocytosis of apoptotic cells in diseased SLE mice. J Autoimmun 22, 139–45

Marino, MJ, Conn, PJ (2002) Direct and indirect modulation of the N-methyl-D-aspartate receptor. Curr Drug Targets CNS Neurol Disord 1, 1–16

Martin, R, Gran, B, Zhao, Y, Markovic-Plese, S, Bielekova, B, Marques, A, Sung, MH, Hemmer, B, Simon, R, McFarland, HF, Pinilla, C (2001) Molecular mimicry and antigen-specific T cell responses in multiple sclerosis and chronic CNS Lyme disease. J Autoimmun 16, 187–92

Mattson, MP, LaFerla, FM, Chan, SL, Leissring, MA, Shepel, PN, Geiger, JD (2000) Calcium signaling in the ER: its role in neuronal plasticity and neurodegenerative disorders. Trends Neurosci 23, 222–9

Morris, RG, Anderson, E, Lynch, GS, Baudry, M (1986) Selective impairment of learning and blockade of long-term potentiation by an N-methyl-D-aspartate receptor antagonist, AP5. Nature 319, 774–6

Oztas, B (1998) Sex and blood-brain barrier. Pharmacol Res 37, 165–7

Oztas, B, Akgul, S, Arslan, FB (2004) Influence of surgical pain stress on the blood-brain barrier permeability in rats. Life Sci 74, 1973–9

Pardridge, W (1998) Introduction to the Blood-Brain Barrier: Methodology, Biology, and Pathology (W. Pardridge, ed.) Cambridge University Press, Cambridge

Paul, R, Lorenzl, S, Koedel, U, Sporer, B, Vogel, U, Frosch, M, Pfister, HW (1998) Matrix metalloproteinases contribute to the blood-brain barrier disruption during bacterial meningitis. Ann Neurol 44, 592–600

Potter, PK, Cortes-Hernandez, J, Quartier, P, Botto, M, Walport, MJ (2003) Lupus-prone mice have an abnormal response to thioglycolate and an impaired clearance of apoptotic cells. J Immunol 170, 3223–32

Putterman, C, Diamond, B (1998) Immunization with a peptide surrogate for double-stranded DNA (dsDNA) induces autoantibody production and renal immunoglobulin deposition. J Exp Med 188, 29–38

Ring, A, Weiser, JN, Tuomanen, EI (1998) Pneumococcal trafficking across the blood-brain barrier. Molecular analysis of a novel bidirectional pathway. J Clin Invest 102, 347–60

Rutter, JV, Jehanli, A, Harrison, R, Lunt, GG (1987) Immunological factors in neuronal degeneration with particular reference to motor neurone disease. Gerontology 33, 187–92

Rutter, M, Schopler, E (1987) Autism and pervasive developmental disorders: concepts and diagnostic issues. J Autism Dev Disord 17, 159–86

Sabbaga, J, Line, SR, Potocnjak, P, Madaio, MP (1989) A murine nephritogenic monoclonal anti-DNA autoantibody binds directly to mouse laminin, the major non-collagenous protein component of the glomerular basement membrane. Eur J Immunol 19, 137–43

Sakic, B, Szechtman, H, Keffer, M, Talangbayan, H, Stead, R, Denburg, JA (1992) A behavioral profile of autoimmune lupus-prone MRL mice. Brain Behav Immun 6, 265–85

Sakic, B, Kolb, B, Whishaw, IQ, Gorny, G, Szechtman, H, Denburg, JA (2000) Immunosuppression prevents neuronal atrophy in lupus-prone mice: evidence for brain damage induced by autoimmune disease? J Neuroimmunol 111, 93–101

Sastre-Garriga, J, Montalban, X (2003) APS and the brain. Lupus 12, 877–82

Scherzer, CR, Landwehrmeyer, GB, Kerner, JA, Counihan, TJ, Kosinski, CM, Standaert, DG, Daggett, LP, Velicelebi, G, Penney, JB, Young, AB (1998) Expression of N-methyl-D-aspartate receptor subunit mRNAs in the human brain: hippocampus and cortex. J Comp Neurol 390, 75–90

Schutzer, SE, Brunner, M, Fillit, HM, Berger, JR (2003) Autoimmune markers in HIV-associated dementia. J Neuroimmunol 138, 156–61

Sherman, GF, Morrison, L, Rosen, GD, Behan, PO, Galaburda, AM (1990) Brain abnormalities in immune defective mice. Brain Res 532, 25–33

Sinha, S, Newsom-Davis, J, Mills, K, Byrne, N, Lang, B, Vincent, A (1991) Autoimmune aetiology for acquired neuromyotonia (Isaacs' syndrome) Lancet 338, 75–7

Staines, DR (2004a) Is fibromyalgia an autoimmune disorder of endogenous vasoactive neuropeptides? Med Hypotheses 62, 665–9

Staines, DR (2004b) Is Gulf War Syndrome an autoimmune disorder of endogenous neuropeptides, exogenous sandfly maxadilan and molecular mimicry? Med Hypotheses 62, 658–64

Staines, DR (2004c) Is sudden infant death syndrome (SIDS) an autoimmune disorder of endogenous vasoactive neuropeptides? Med Hypotheses 62, 653–7

Standaert, DG, Testa, CM, Young, AB, Penney, JB, Jr (1994) Organization of *N*-methyl-D-aspartate glutamate receptor gene expression in the basal ganglia of the rat. J Comp Neurol 343, 1–16

Stein, CM, Olson, JM, Gray-McGuire, C, Bruner, GR, Harley, JB, Moser, KL (2002) Increased prevalence of renal disease in systemic lupus erythematosus families with affected male relatives. Arthritis Rheum 46, 428–35

Szechtman, H, Sakic, B, Denburg, JA (1997) Behaviour of MRL mice: an animal model of disturbed behaviour in systemic autoimmune disease. Lupus 6, 223–9

Tanaka, S, Kuratsune, H, Hidaka, Y, Hakariya, Y, Tatsumi, KI, Takano, T, Kanakura, Y, Amino, N (2003) Autoantibodies against muscarinic cholinergic receptor in chronic fatigue syndrome. Int J Mol Med 12, 225–30

Trivedi, DH, Bussel, JB (2003) 21. Immunohematologic disorders. J Allergy Clin Immunol 111, S669–76

Venkatesh, J, Diamond, B (2004) Unpublished observations

Vojdani, A, Campbell, AW, Anyanwu, E, Kashanian, A, Bock, K, Vojdani, E (2002) Antibodies to neuron-specific antigens in children with autism: possible cross-reaction with encephalitogenic proteins from milk, *Chlamydia pneumoniae* and *Streptococcus* group A. J Neuroimmunol 129, 168–77

Waterhouse, DM, Natale, RB, Cody, RL (1991) Breast cancer and paraneoplastic cerebellar degeneration. Cancer 68, 1835–41

Xaio, H, Banks, WA, Niehoff, ML, Morley, JE (2001) Effect of LPS on the permeability of the blood-brain barrier to insulin. Brain Res 896, 36–42

Chlamydia and Antigenic Mimicry

K. Bachmaier[1] (✉) · J. M. Penninger[2]

[1]Department of Pharmacology, College of Medicine, University of Illinois at Chicago, E403, Medical Sciences Building, M/C 868, 835 S. Wolcott Avenue, Chicago, IL 60612, USA

[2]IMBA, Institute for Molecular Biotechnology of the Austrian Academy of Sciences, Dr Bohr Gasse 3-5, 1030 Vienna, Austria
kbachmai@uic.edu

1	Chlamydial Proteins That Mimic Endogenous Proteins	154
1.1	Chlamydial Hsp60	155
1.2	DNA Primase of *Chlamydia trachomatis*	155
1.3	*Chlamydia* OmcB Proteins	156
2	Molecular Mimicry of Endogenous Proteins by Chlamydial Proteins and Human Disease	158
2.1	Atherosclerosis	158
2.2	Arthritis	159
2.3	Pelvic Inflammatory Disease	160
2.4	Dilated Cardiomyopathy	160
3	Conclusions	161
References		161

Abstract Chlamydial infections are among the most common human infections. Every year, in millions of humans, they cause infections of the eyes, the respiratory tract, the genital tract, joints, and the vasculature. *Chlamydiae* are obligate intracellular prokaryotic pathogens. *Chlamydiae* promote, in susceptible host cells that include mucosal epithelial cells, vascular endothelial cells, smooth muscle cells, and monocytes and macrophages, their survival while causing disease of varying clinical importance and consequence in their hosts. *Chlamydia* infections often precede the initiation of autoimmune diseases, and *Chlamydiae* are often found within autoimmune lesions. Thus, they have been suspected in the etiology and pathogenesis of autoimmune diseases. Autoimmune diseases have many causes. Genes, notably genes encoding cell-surface proteins that display peptides for immune recognition, the major histocompatibility complex (MHC), the environment, and the microbial diversity within the human body determine the susceptibility to autoimmune diseases. One mechanism by which infection is linked to the initiation of autoimmunity is termed molecular mimicry. Molecular mimicry describes the phenomenon of protein products from dissimilar genes sharing similar structures that elicit an immune response to both self and microbial proteins. Molecular mimicry might thus be a mechanism by which infections trigger autoimmune diseases. For the purpose of this chapter, we will focus on chlamydial proteins that mimic host self-proteins and thus contribute to initiation and maintenance of autoimmune diseases. Thus far, the strongest cases for molecular mimicry seem to have been made for chlamydial heat shock proteins 60, the DNA primase of *Chlamydia trachomatis*, and chlamydial OmcB proteins.

> What bacteria do is of very much more moment than what they look like.
>
> Macfarlane Burnett

1
Chlamydial Proteins That Mimic Endogenous Proteins

There is ample evidence that in the pathogenesis of many important human diseases, cellular and humoral immune response are directed at self-proteins (Rose and Mackay 1985). What is less clear is the etiology of such autoimmune responses. However, there is epidemiological, clinical, and experimental evidence of associations between autoimmunity and infection. Indeed, the first autoimmune diseases to be described, early in the twentieth century, were sequelae of infections (Silverstein 2001). Molecular mimicry describes the phenomenon of protein products from dissimilar genes, for example, proteins derived from microbes and humans, sharing similar structures that elicit cross-reactivity of the adaptive immune system with host self and microbial epitopes (Oldstone 1987). Molecular mimicry might thus be a mechanism by which infections trigger autoimmune diseases. Criteria to judge molecular mimicry as a mechanism by which infection triggers autoimmunity should contain: The responsible epitopes, from microbial and self-proteins, should be known. The microbial epitope should be able to elicit a lymphocyte response that is cross-reactive to the self-epitope. The relevance of the microbial and self-epitopes, and the cross-reactive response to them, needs to be established. For example, can antigen-presenting cells that display mimicking epitopes be found in autoimmune lesions? Do cross-reactive lymphocytes expand during the immune response that triggers disease? Are both, microbial and self-epitopes, necessary for the development of the autoimmune disease? It is important to stringently distinguish between a mechanism that involves molecular mimicry and other, diverse mechanisms (Benoist and Mathis 2001). According to these criteria the current examples for molecular mimicry caused by chlamydial proteins will be examined. For the purpose of this chapter, we will focus on chlamydial proteins that mimic host self-proteins and thus contribute to initiation and maintenance of autoimmune diseases. The strongest cases for molecular mimicry have been made for chlamydial heat shock proteins 60, the DNA primase of *Chlamydia trachomatis*, and chlamydial OmcB proteins.

1.1
Chlamydial Hsp60

Heat shock proteins (hsp) are produced by cells in response to, for example, an increase in temperature, cytokines, or free radicals. Hsp are evolutionary conserved, having a high degree of amino acid sequence homology among all species, ranging from prokaryotes to humans. Mouse hsp60 and hsp60 from *Chlamydia trachomatis* share a high degree of amino acid sequence identity. Attempts to induce autoimmunity using endogenous and chlamydial Hsp60 proteins in mice showed that autoimmune responses were induced only by immunization with both mouse and chlamydial hsp60 proteins. Immunization with mouse hsp60 alone induced T lymphocytes that secreted high levels of interleukin-10 (IL10) but did not proliferate in response to in vitro stimulation with mouse hsp60. On the other hand, co-immunization with mouse and chlamydial hsp60s induced T lymphocytes that proliferated strongly in response to mouse hsp60, and secreted high levels of interferon gamma (IFNγ) and low levels of IL10 (Yi et al. 1997). These results, while consistent with the notion of molecular mimicry, do not actually prove it. T cells reactive to chlamydial hsp60 following experimental murine infection have been described by others as well (Beatty and Stephens 1992); however, whether these T cells would react to endogenous hsp60 was not addressed. Similarly, T cells obtained from *Chlamydia*-infected patients that were specific for chlamydial hsp60 were not tested for cross-reactivity to human hsp60 (Witkin et al. 1994; Kinnunen et al. 2002). These human T cells predominantly produced IL10, (Kinnunen et al. 2002), a cytokine that would downregulate Th1-mediated immune responses. IL10, a cytokine that inhibits IFNγ production and that is restricted, in mice, to Th2 cells, predominates in murine models of chlamydial infection (Yang et al. 1999; Morrison and Morrison 2000; Yi et al. 1997). Others have shown that T-cell lines, established from atherosclerotic plaques of carotid artery tissue specimens obtained from patients who had undergone carotid endarterectomy, proliferated to stimulation with chlamydial hsp60 (Mosorin et al. 2000). However, cross-reactivity to endogenous hsp60 was not tested.

1.2
DNA Primase of *Chlamydia trachomatis*

HLA-B27 is strongly associated with spondyloarthropathies, including ankylosing spondylitis and reactive arthritis. It has been proposed that presentation by HLA-B27 of peptides derived from its own molecule with homology to bacterial proteins could be responsible for autoimmunity following bacterial infection. Ramos et al. demonstrated that a 12-amino acid peptide derived from the intracytoplasmic tail of HLA-B27, corresponding to amino-acid residues 309–320, RRKSSGGKGGSY, was a natural ligand, in vivo, of three disease-associated subtypes (B*2702, B*2704, and B*2705) but not of two (B*2706 and B*2709) that are only weakly or not associated with spondyloarthropathy. A homologous synthetic peptide derived the DNA primase of *Chlamydia trachomatis,* aa211–222: RRFKEGGRGGKY, bound, *in vitro,* disease-associated subtypes equally well as the natural B27-derived ligand. Molecular modeling suggested that the B27-derived and chlamydial peptides take on very similar conformations in complex with B*2705. Interestingly, this chlamydial peptide was generated following proteolysis by the 20S proteasome, the major proteinase generating antigenic peptides in cells. The results demonstrate that an HLA-B27-derived peptide and mimicking chlamydial peptides are natural ligands of disease-associated HLA-B27 subtypes (Ramos et al. 2002). Furthermore, HLA-B27-mimicking chlamydial peptide might be presented by HLA-B27 on *Chlamydia*-infected cells and thus have etiologic and pathogenetic roles in reactive arthritis.

1.3
Chlamydia OmcB Proteins

In vivo mapping of a pathogenic motif, first discovered on endogenous α-myosin heavy chain protein, was used to directly test the mechanism of molecular mimicry (Bachmaier et al. 1999). In mice, immunization with heart muscle myosin induces autoimmune myocarditis (Neu et al. 1987), a disease that is dependent on $CD4^+$ T cells that recognize a heart muscle-specific peptide in association with self major histocompatibility complex (MHC) class II molecules. The identification of pathogenic epitopes on the myosin molecule was based on the comparison of the pathogenicity between cardiac α-myosin and soleus muscle β-myosin. Only α-myosin was found to induce myocarditis, with high severity and prevalence (Pummerer et al. 1996). Therefore, the epitopes present on immunodominant α-myosin but absent in the nonpathogenic β-myosin were synthesized and tested for their ability to induce inflammatory heart disease. Thus, pathogenic epitopes on the murine heart muscle-specific α-myosin heavy chain were identified (Pummerer et al. 1996). Immunization with a 16-amino acid peptide, aa614–629: SLKLMATLF-STYASAD, of the cardiac-specific α-myosin heavy chain, designated M7Aα, induces severe inflammatory heart disease in BALB/c mice (Table 1) (Bachmaier et al. 1999). In contrast, the homologous region of the β-myosin heavy chain isoform (M7Aβ) which contains defined amino acid changes does not induce disease (Table 1). The introduction of single amino acid substitutions into M7Aα further revealed that the residues xxxMAxxxSTxxx were important for the pathogenicity of M7Aα in vivo. These immunogenic amino acids are conserved between murine and human α-myosin heavy chains, and injection of the human M7Aα homologue into BALB/c mice induces inflammatory heart disease (K. Bachmaier, unpublished data). To test whether the *Chlamydia* peptides containing the M7Aα motif could induce inflammatory heart disease, BALB/c mice were immunized with murine M7Aα or the homologous peptides, derived from the OmcB proteins of *Chlamydia trachomatis*, *Chlamydia psittaci*, and *Chlamydia pneumoniae*. All were able to induce inflammatory heart disease at a similar frequency, albeit at significantly lower severity, as compared to M7Aα-immunized mice (Table 1). Like the inflammation that follows immunization with the endogenous autoantigen M7Aα, the disease induced by all the *Chlamydia*-derived peptides was characterized by perivascular and pericardial infiltration of mononuclear cells and fibrotic changes. These results suggested that antigenic mimicry between *Chlamydia* peptides and a heart muscle-specific myosin peptide can lead to the development of inflammatory heart disease. To directly address the hypothesis of antigenic mimicry between an endogenous cardiac-specific peptide and *Chlamydia*-derived peptides, T cell proliferation studies were performed. T cells from mice immunized with the endogenous peptide M7Aα strongly proliferated when incubated with splenocytes pulsed with the M7Aα peptide. T cells from these mice also showed a strong proliferative response to the *Chlamydia*-derived peptide (Bachmaier et al. 1999). Importantly, splenic T cells from mice immunized with *Chlamydia*-derived peptide proliferated strongly against *Chlamydia*-derived peptide as well as against the endogenous M7Aα peptide. These data demonstrated that *Chlamydia*-derived peptide

Table 1 Sequence alignment of chlamydial peptides with the pathogenic mouse M7Aα and the non-pathogenic mouse M7Aβ peptides

Peptide	Amino acid sequence	Prevalence	Severity
M7Aα	SLKLMATLFSTYASA	High	Severe
Chlamydia trachomatis	VLETSMAEFTSTNVIS	High	Mild
Chlamydia trachomatis	VLETSMAESLSTNVIS	High	Mild
Chlamydia pneumoniae	GIEAAVAESLITKIVA	High	Mild
Chlamydia psittaci	KIEAAAAESLATRFIA	Low	Mild
M7Aβ	SLKLLSNLFANYASA	–	–

immunizations can crossprime for T cell reactivity against the endogenous M7Aα. Immunization with endogenous M7Aα peptide led to the production of serum antibodies reactive against the M7Aα peptide used for the induction of the disease. Mice immunized with the endogenous peptide M7Aα also showed serum antibodies reactive against the *Chlamydia*-derived peptide. Likewise, immunization with *Chlamydia*-derived peptide induced the production of serum antibodies reactive against the endogenous M7Aα. The peptides used in these studies are located within the leader signal peptide of OmcB proteins (Allen and Stephens 1989). Thus, these peptides might be cleaved from the mature protein during translocation and, degraded, be unavailable to elicit antibody responses during a natural infection. However, actual *Chlamydia* infections lead to the activation of autoaggressive lymphocytes reactive to heart-specific antigens. BALB/c mice were infected with *Chlamydia trachomatis* through the respiratory tract and the reproductive organs. Chlamydial infection led to the production of IgG antibodies to heart-specific epitopes in BALB/c mice (Bachmaier et al. 1999). These data demonstrated that infection by *Chlamydia trachomatis* activates autoaggressive lymphocytes in BALB/c mice. Thus, *Chlamydia*-mediated heart disease in mice is induced by antigenic mimicry of a heart muscle-specific protein.

2
Molecular Mimicry of Endogenous Proteins by Chlamydial Proteins and Human Disease

There is ample evidence that many important human diseases, leading causes of illness and death, are linked to infectious agents. In the sections that follow, the case for autoimmunity, and of molecular mimicry as its inducing mechanism, is presented for atherosclerosis, arthritis, pelvic inflammatory disease, and dilated cardiomyopathy.

2.1
Atherosclerosis

Cardiovascular disease is the leading cause of death and illness in rich countries and predictions are that it will soon become the pre-eminent disease worldwide (Murray and Lopez 1997). Atherosclerosis, the single most important contributor to this growing health care burden, is a progressive disease characterized by an ongoing inflammatory response and the accumulation of lipids and fibrous elements in the large arteries. Infection with *Chlamydia pneumoniae* is an emerging risk factor for cardiovascular disease. *Chlamydiae* produce large amounts of hsp60 during chronic, persistent infections.

Atherosclerotic lesions often contain chlamydial and human hsp60. Both stimulate macrophage functions, in a manner relevant to atherosclerosis and its complications, such as production of proinflammatory cytokines, TNFα, and matrix-degrading metalloproteinases (Kol et al. 1998). Whether chlamydial hsp60 might mediate the induction of these effects by mimicking endogenous hsp60 has, however, not been tested. Serum reactivity to the chlamydial hsp60 is an independent risk factor, but, according to one study, specifically independent of reactivity to human hsp60. The presence of elevated anti-chlamydial hsp60 IgG antibodies, but not anti-human or anti-*E. coli* homologues, is independently associated with coronary artery disease (Mahdi et al. 2002). On the other hand, high anti-chlamydial hsp60 antibody response might identify a subset of patients with chlamydial infection and significant coronary artery disease (Mahdi et al. 2002). In a more recent study, high levels of antibodies to human hsp60, among patients with antibody levels to *Chlamydia pneumoniae*, was shown to represent independent risk factors for the development of acute myocardial infarction (Heltai et al. 2004). There are, as mentioned previously, human T-cell lines, established from atherosclerotic plaques, that proliferated to stimulation with chlamydial hsp60 (Mosorin et al. 2000). Again, it is not clear whether molecular mimicry is responsible for this effect, since molecular mimicry has not been tested. At this point, there is not enough evidence unequivocally linking autoimmunity to endogenous hsp60, or the mechanism of molecular mimicry, etiology, and pathogenesis of atherosclerosis (Stephens 2003).

2.2
Arthritis

Reactive arthritis can be triggered by infections of the urogenital tract with *Chlamydia trachomatis* (Keat et al. 1987; Braun et al. 1995), and chlamydia-induced arthritis is the most frequent form of reactive arthritis in Western countries (Zeidler et al. 2004). There is some evidence of involvement of autoimmunity in the course of oligoarticular juvenile rheumatoid arthritis: T lymphocytes react to endogenous human hsp60. It is noteworthy, however, that T cell reactivity to human hsp60 was associated with disease remission (Prakken et al. 1996). No evidence exists to implicate molecular mimicry in the pathogenesis of juvenile rheumatoid arthritis. HLA-B27 is strongly associated with spondyloarthropathies, including ankylosing spondylitis and reactive arthritis. Recently, it was demonstrated that HLA-B27 binds in vivo a peptide from its own molecule, B27(309–320). B27(309–320) is a natural ligand of arthritis-associated subtypes, but not of subtypes weakly or not associated to this disease. Thus, among known HLA-B27 ligands derived from the B27 molecule itself, this peptide shows the best correlation with association to ankylosing spondylitis. The homologous chlamydial peptide DNA primase (211–222) binds in vitro B*2702, B*2704, and B*2705 with the same efficiency as the B27-derived peptide, suggesting that, if generated in vivo, this bacterial peptide could be presented by these three subtypes on *Chlamydia*-infected cells. Moreover, chlamydial peptide was generated following proteolysis by the 20S proteasome, the major proteinase generating antigenic peptides in cells. The results demonstrate that an HLA-B27-derived peptide and mimicking chlamydial peptides are natural ligands of disease-associated HLA-B27 subtypes (Ramos et al. 2002). These finding might provide a molecular basis for the association between *Chlamydia* and arthritis. However, this work does not explain why only a very small proportion of HLA-B27-positive individuals develop disease.

2.3
Pelvic Inflammatory Disease

Pelvic inflammatory disease is an infection of the upper female genital tract encompassing endometritis, parametritis, salpingitis, oophoritis, and peritonitis. Complications include infertility, ectopic pregnancy, and chronic pain. Serum antibodies to chlamydial hsp60 are associated with an increased risk for pelvic inflammatory disease caused by infection with *Chlamydia trachomatis* (Peeling et al. 1997). When the serum reactivity to chlamydial hsp60 antigen, among women with high antibody titers to *Chlamydia trachomatis*, was assessed, 80% of the sera from women with ectopic pregnancy, a severe consequence of *Chlamydia trachomatis* infection, showed reactivity, compared to only 31% of sera obtained from women with salpingitis (Wagar et al. 1990; Cerrone et al. 1991). These findings link serum reactivity to *Chlamydia trachomatis* hsp60 to severe disease outcomes. The issue of whether chlamydial pelvic inflammatory disease is a consequence of persistent infection, immunopathology, or molecular mimicry remains unresolved.

2.4
Dilated Cardiomyopathy

Dilated cardiomyopathy (DCM) is the prime condition that necessitates heart transplantations. Approximately 50% of DCM is caused by inflammation of the myocardium. Myocarditis and DCM are closely mimicked by the experimental inflammatory heart disease in mice. Experimental models demonstrating that the *Chlamydia*-derived peptides can cause myocarditis in mice—and that natural infection with both *Chlamydia pneumoniae* (Blessing et al. 2000) and *Chlamydia trachomatis* (Fan et al. 1999) leads to inflammatory heart disease similar to the one seen after immunization with *Chlamydia*-derived peptides—suggest the possibility of molecular mimicry in the etiology and pathogenesis of human inflammatory heart disease. In humans, *Chlamydia trachomatis* infections have been directly linked to myocarditis (Odeh et al. 1991; Grayston et al. 1981; Wesslen et al. 1992; Tong et al. 1995). Furthermore, there is now the first clinical evidence that DCM in patients is associated with persistent *Chlamydia pneumoniae* infection (Song et al. 2001). Conclusive evidence for molecular mimicry in human DCM is still lacking.

3
Conclusions

Criteria have been designed to stringently distinguish between a mechanism that involves molecular mimicry and other, diverse mechanisms. Rational treatment strategies for disease rely on a correct understanding of the etiology and pathogenesis of these diseases. Associations between a particular microbial infection and a particular inflammatory state are numerous. Disease-causing microbial and self-proteins have been identified. In many cases, the relevance of the microbial and self-epitopes for human disease remains unclear. As for *Chlamydiae*, it seems fair to say that the case for molecular mimicry is still open. Where the experimental evidence for molecular mimicry is strong, the clinical and epidemiological evidence is weak. Where the epidemiological and clinical evidence is ample, the experimental support is weak. Unless we continue to gain further insights in the etiology and pathogenesis of *Chlamydia*-associated diseases, we will not be able to devise better treatment strategies for some of the most important human diseases.

Acknowledgements We thank L.A. Benoit, C. Richardson, T. Wada, N. Neu for helpful comments and advice.

References

Allen J E, Stephens RS (1989) Identification by Sequence-analysis of 2-site posttranslational processing of the cysteine-rich outer-membrane protein-2 of *Chlamydia trachomatis* serovar-L2. J Bacteriol171:285–291

Bachmaier K, Neu N, de la Maza LM, Pal S, Hessel A, Penninger JM (1999) Chlamydia infections and heart disease linked through antigenic mimicry. Science 283:1335–1339

Beatty PR, Stephens RS (1992) Identification of *Chlamydia trachomatis* antigens by use of murine T-cell lines. Infect Immun 60:4598–4603

Benoist C, Mathis D (2001) Autoimmunity provoked by infection: how good is the case for T cell epitope mimicry? Nat Immunol 2:797–801

Blessing E, Lin TM, Campbell LA, Rosenfeld ME, Lloyd D, Kuo CC (2000) *Chlamydia pneumoniae* induces inflammatory changes in the heart and aorta of normocholesterolemic C57BL/6J mice. Infect Immun 68:4765–4768

Braun J, Laitko S, Treharne J, Eggens U, Wu PH, Distler A, Sieper J (1994) *Chlamydia pneumoniae*—a new causative agent of reactive arthritis and undifferentiated oligoarthritis. Ann Rheum Dis 53:100–105

Cerrone MC, Ma JJ, Stephens RS (1991) Cloning and sequence of the gene for heat-shock protein-60 from *Chlamydia trachomatis* and immunological reactivity of the protein. Infect Immun 59:79–90

Fan YJ, Wang SH, Yang X (1999) *Chlamydia trachomatis* (Mouse pneumonitis strain) induces cardiovascular pathology following respiratory tract infection. Infect Immun 67:6145–6151

Grayston JT, Mordhorst CH, Wang SP (1981) Childhood myocarditis associated with *Chlamydia trachomatis* infection. JAMA 246:2823–2827

Heltai K, Kis Z, Burian K, Endresz V, Veres A, Ludwig E, Gonczol E, Valyi-Nagy I (2004) Elevated antibody levels against *Chlamydia pneumoniae*, human HSP60 and mycobacterial HSP65 are independent risk factors in myocardial infarction and ischaemic heart disease. Atherosclerosis 173:339–346

Keat A, Dixey J, Sonnex C, Thomas B, Osborn M, Taylorrobinson, D (1987) *Chlamydia trachomatis* and reactive arthritis—the missing link. Lancet 1:72–74

Kinnunen A, Molander P, Morrison R, Lehtinen M, Karttunen R, Tiitinen A, Paavonen J, Surcel HM (2002) Chlamydial heat shock protein 60-specific T cells in inflamed salpingeal tissue. Fertil Steril 77:162–166

Kol A, Sukhova GK, Lichtman AH, Libby P (1998) Chlamydial heat shock protein 60 localizes in human atheroma and regulates macrophage tumor necrosis factor-alpha and matrix metalloproteinase expression. Circulation 98:300–307

Mahdi OS, Horne BD, Mullen K, Muhlestein JB, Byrne GI (2002) Serum immunoglobulin g antibodies to chlamydial heat shock protein 60 but not to human and bacterial homologs are associated with coronary artery disease. Circulation 106:1659–1663

Morrison SG, Morrison RP (2000) In situ analysis of the evolution of the primary immune response in murine *Chlamydia trachomatis* genital tract infection. Infection and Immunity 68:2870–2879

Mosorin M, Surcel HM, Laurila A, Lehtinen M, Karttunen R, Juvonen J, Paavonen J, Morrison RP, Saikku P, Juvonen T (2000) Detection of *Chlamydia pneumoniae*-reactive T lymphocytes in human atherosclerotic plaques of carotid artery. Arterioscler Thromb Vasc Biol 20:1061–1067

Murray CJL, Lopez AD (1997) Global mortality, disability, and the contribution of risk factors: Global Burden of Disease Study. Lancet 349:1436–1442

Neu N, Rose NR, Beisel KW, Herskowitz A, Gurriglass G, Craig SW (1987) Cardiac myosin induces myocarditis in genetically predisposed mice. J Immunol 139:3630–3636

Odeh M, Oliven A (1992) Chlamydial infections of the heart. Eur J Clin Microbiol Infect Dis 11:885–893

Oldstone MBA (1987) Molecular mimicry and autoimmune disease. Cell 50:819–820

Peeling RW, Kimani J, Plummer F, Maclean I, Cheang M, Bwayo J, Brunham RC (1997) Antibody to chlamydial hsp60 predicts an increased risk for chlamydial pelvic inflammatory disease. J Infect Dis 175:1153–1158

Prakken ABJ, vanEden W, Rijkers GT, Kuis W, Toebes EA, DeGraeffMeeder ER, vanderZee R, Zegers BJM (1996) Autoreactivity to human heat-shock protein 60 predicts disease remission in oligoarticular juvenile rheumatoid arthritis. Arthrit Rheumat 39:1826–1832

Pummerer CL, Luze K, Grassl G, Bachmaier K, Offner F, Burrell SK, Lenz DM, Zamborelli TJ, Penninger JM, Neu N (1996) Identification of cardiac myosin peptides capable of inducing autoimmune myocarditis in BALB/c mice. J Clin Invest 97:2057–2062

Ramos M, Alvarez I, Sesma L, Logean A, Rognan D, de Castro JAL (2002) Molecular mimicry of an HLA-B27-derived ligand of arthritis-linked subtypes with chlamydial proteins. J Biol Chem 277:37573–37581

Rose NR, Mackay IR (eds) (1985) *The Autoimmune Diseases* p. iv (New York, Academic Press)

Silverstein AM (2001) Autoimmunity versus horror autotoxicus: the struggle for recognition. Nat Immunol 2:279–281

Song H, Tasaki H, Yashiro A, Yamashita K, Toyokawa T, Nagai Y, Takatsu H, Taniguchi H, Nakashima Y (2001) Dilated cardiomyopathy and *Chlamydia pneumoniae* infection. Heart 86:456–456

Stephens RS (2003) The cellular paradigm of chlamydial pathogenesis. Trends Microbiol 11:44–51

Tong CYW, Potter F, Worthington E, Mullins P (1995) *Chlamydia pneumoniae* myocarditis. Lancet 346:710–711

Wagar EA, Schachter J, Bavoil P, Stephens RS (1990) Differential human serologic response to 2 60,000 molecular-weight *Chlamydia trachomatis* antigens. J Infect Dis 162:922–927

Wesslen L, Pahlson C, Friman G, Fohlman J, Lindquist O, Johansson C (1992) Myocarditis caused by *Chlamydia pneumoniae* (Twar) and sudden unexpected death in a Swedish elite orienteer. Lancet 340:427–428

Witkin SS, Jeremias J, Toth M, Ledger WJ (1994) Proliferative response to conserved epitopes of the *Chlamydia trachomatis* and human 60-kilodalton heat-shock proteins by lymphocytes from women with salpingitis. Am J Obstet Gynecol 171:455–460

Yang X, Gartner J, Zhu LH, Wang SH, Brunham RC (1999) IL-10 gene knockout mice show enhanced Th1-like protective immunity and absent granuloma formation following *Chlamydia trachomatis* lung infection. J Immunol 162:1010–1017

Yi YJ, Yang X, Brunham RC (1997) Autoimmunity to heat shock protein 60 and antigen-specific production of interleukin-10. Infect Immun 65:1669–1674

Yi YJ, Zhong GM, Brunham RC (1993). Continuous B-cell epitopes in *Chlamydia trachomatis* heat-shock protein-60. Infect Immun 61:1117–1120

Zeidler H, Kuipers J, Kohler L (2004) *Chlamydia*-induced arthritis. Curr Opin Rheumatol 16:380–392

Subject Index

alpha actinin 140
amygdala 146
anti-DNA antibodies 138–141, 143
anti-dsDNA antibodies 141
antigen presenting cells (APC)
- bystander activation 108
- cryptic epitopes presented by 98
antigen-presenting cells 48, 154
anti-pneumococcal antibodies 139
apoptosis 144, 145
apoptotic cells 138
apoptotic debris 139
autoimmune disease 39

BALB/c 156–158
BBB 142, 144–146
Betz cells 129, 132
blood-brain barrier 142
BRAAs 142, 143
brain-reactive autoantibodies (BRAAs) 141
bystander activation 41

$CD4^+$ cells
- $CD4^+$ T cell line 106
- delayed-hypersensitivity (DTH) type 95
- infiltration by 94
$CD4^+$ T cells 39
$CD8^+$ cells
- T cruzi infection 93
central nervous system 42, 125, 138
cerebrospinal fluid 40
chronic inflammation 95
corticospinal 126, 129, 131, 132

cross-reactive $CD4^+$ T cell response 44
cross-reactivities 140
CTL 93
cytokines
- bystander activation 108
- induction of adhesion molecules 96
- protective response 93

demyelinating disease 39

epinephrine 144, 146
epitope 128, 130

haemophilus influenzae 39
heparan sulfate 140
heterogeneous nuclear ribonuclear protein A1 125
hippocampal 143, 145
hippocampus 143–146
HLA-B27 155, 156, 159, 160
hnRNP A1 131–133
hnRNP A2 133
HTLV-1-associated myelopathy/tropical spastic paraparesis 125, 126
HTLV-1-*env* and *tax* 127
human histocompatibility leukocyte antigen 126
human histocompatibility leukocyte antigen (HLA) DRB*10101 125
human T-lymphotropic virus type 1 125, 126

IFN-γ   93, 109
immunization   155, 156, 158, 161
immunodominant   125, 127, 128, 130, 132
immunodominant epitope   131
immunoglobulins   127
inflammation
– cardiac   107
– cardiomyocyte damage   102
– chronic   94
iNOS   93, 102
interferon (IFN)γ   155
interleukin (IL)10   155

laminin   140
lipopolysaccharide   144
LPS   145

magnetic resonance spectroscopy   145
major histocompatibility complex (MHC)   90
mass spectroscopy   129
memantine   145
memory   141, 143, 145
meningoencephalitis   91
MHC   153, 156
microbial antigen   139, 140
microbial antigens   139
microglial cell   42
Mimotope   130
MK-801   144
molecular mimicry   39, 138, 139, 142
motor   126, 129, 130, 132
multiple sclerosis   39, 125
myelin   39
myelin oligodendrocyte glycoprotein   41
myocardial infarction   159, 162
Myosin   156
myosin   157

N-acetyl aspartate (NAA)   145
neuronal apoptosis   143

neuronal damage   95, 96
neuronal death   138
neurons   138
neuropsychiatric symptoms   142
NMDA   141
NMDA receptor antagonist MK801   143
NMDA receptors   138, 145

patch-clamp   130
peptide   140, 141, 144
phage peptide display library   140
pneumococcal cell wall polysaccharide   139
pneumococcal choline kinase   140
pneumococcal polysaccharide   139
polyclonal lymphocyte activation   98
proteolipid protein   41

recombinant TMEV   42
renal antigens   140

self-proteins   154, 161
seronegative   128, 129
symptoms   138, 142
systemic lupus erythematosus   138

T cells   155
T-cell leukemia   126
Theiler's murine encephalomyelitis virus   39
TNF   98
TNFα   159
tolerance   42
trypanosoma cruzi   91
– immune response   93
– life cycle   91
– transmission   91

viral load   126, 128
virus infection   42

Current Topics in Microbiology and Immunology

Volumes published since 1989 (and still available)

Vol. 251: **Melchers, Fritz (Ed.):** Lymphoid Organogenesis. 2000. 62 figs. XII, 215 pp. ISBN 3-540-67569-8

Vol. 252: **Potter, Michael; Melchers, Fritz (Eds.):** B1 Lymphocytes in B Cell Neoplasia. 2000. XIII, 326 pp. ISBN 3-540-67567-1

Vol. 253: **Gosztonyi, Georg (Ed.):** The Mechanisms of Neuronal Damage in Virus Infections of the Nervous System. 2001. approx. XVI, 270 pp. ISBN 3-540-67617-1

Vol. 254: **Privalsky, Martin L. (Ed.):** Transcriptional Corepressors. 2001. 25 figs. XIV, 190 pp. ISBN 3-540-67569-8

Vol. 255: **Hirai, Kanji (Ed.):** Marek's Disease. 2001. 22 figs. XII, 294 pp. ISBN 3-540-67798-4

Vol. 256: **Schmaljohn, Connie S.; Nichol, Stuart T. (Eds.):** Hantaviruses. 2001. 24 figs. XI, 196 pp. ISBN 3-540-41045-7

Vol. 257: **van der Goot, Gisou (Ed.):** PoreForming Toxins, 2001. 19 figs. IX, 166 pp. ISBN 3-540-41386-3

Vol. 258: **Takada, Kenzo (Ed.):** Epstein-Barr Virus and Human Cancer. 2001. 38 figs. IX, 233 pp. ISBN 3-540-41506-8

Vol. 259: **Hauber, Joachim, Vogt, Peter K. (Eds.):** Nuclear Export of Viral RNAs. 2001. 19 figs. IX, 131 pp. ISBN 3-540-41278-6

Vol. 260: **Burton, Didier R. (Ed.):** Antibodies in Viral Infection. 2001. 51 figs. IX, 309 pp. ISBN 3-540-41611-0

Vol. 261: **Trono, Didier (Ed.):** Lentiviral Vectors. 2002. 32 figs. X, 258 pp. ISBN 3-540-42190-4

Vol. 262: **Oldstone, Michael B.A. (Ed.):** Arenaviruses I. 2002. 30 figs. XVIII, 197 pp. ISBN 3-540-42244-7

Vol. 263: **Oldstone, Michael B. A. (Ed.):** Arenaviruses II. 2002. 49 figs. XVIII, 268 pp. ISBN 3-540-42705-8

Vol. 264/I: **Hacker, Jörg; Kaper, James B. (Eds.):** Pathogenicity Islands and the Evolution of Microbes. 2002. 34 figs. XVIII, 232 pp. ISBN 3-540-42681-7

Vol. 264/II: **Hacker, Jörg; Kaper, James B. (Eds.):** Pathogenicity Islands and the Evolution of Microbes. 2002. 24 figs. XVIII, 228 pp. ISBN 3-540-42682-5

Vol. 265: **Dietzschold, Bernhard; Richt, Jürgen A. (Eds.):** Protective and Pathological Immune Responses in the CNS. 2002. 21 figs. X, 278 pp. ISBN 3-540-42668X

Vol. 266: **Cooper, Koproski (Eds.):** The Interface Between Innate and Acquired Immunity, 2002. 15 figs. XIV, 116 pp. ISBN 3-540-42894-X

Vol. 267: **Mackenzie, John S.; Barrett, Alan D. T.; Deubel, Vincent (Eds.):** Japanese Encephalitis and West Nile Viruses. 2002. 66 figs. X, 418 pp. ISBN 3-540-42783X

Vol. 268: **Zwickl, Peter; Baumeister, Wolfgang (Eds.):** The Proteasome-Ubiquitin Protein Degradation Pathway. 2002. 17 figs. X, 213 pp. ISBN 3-540-43096-2

Vol. 269: **Koszinowski, Ulrich H.; Hengel, Hartmut (Eds.):** Viral Proteins Counteracting Host Defenses. 2002. 47 figs. XII, 325 pp. ISBN 3-540-43261-2

Vol. 270: **Beutler, Bruce; Wagner, Hermann (Eds.):** Toll-Like Receptor Family Members and Their Ligands. 2002. 31 figs. X, 192 pp. ISBN 3-540-43560-3

Vol. 271: **Koehler, Theresa M. (Ed.):** Anthrax. 2002. 14 figs. X, 169 pp. ISBN 3-540-43497-6

Vol. 272: **Doerfler, Walter; Böhm, Petra (Eds.):** Adenoviruses: Model and Vectors in Virus-Host Interactions. Virion and

Structure, Viral Replication, Host Cell Interactions. 2003. 63 figs., approx. 280 pp. ISBN 3-540-00154-9

Vol. 273: **Doerfler, Walter; Böhm, Petra (Eds.):** Adenoviruses: Model and Vectors in VirusHost Interactions. Immune System, Oncogenesis, Gene Therapy. 2004. 35 figs., approx. 280 pp. ISBN 3-540-06851-1

Vol. 274: **Workman, Jerry L. (Ed.):** Protein Complexes that Modify Chromatin. 2003. 38 figs., XII, 296 pp. ISBN 3-540-44208-1

Vol. 275: **Fan, Hung (Ed.):** Jaagsiekte Sheep Retrovirus and Lung Cancer. 2003. 63 figs., XII, 252 pp. ISBN 3-540-44096-3

Vol. 276: **Steinkasserer, Alexander (Ed.):** Dendritic Cells and Virus Infection. 2003. 24 figs., X, 296 pp. ISBN 3-540-44290-1

Vol. 277: **Rethwilm, Axel (Ed.):** Foamy Viruses. 2003. 40 figs., X, 214 pp. ISBN 3-540-44388-6

Vol. 278: **Salomon, Daniel R.; Wilson, Carolyn (Eds.):** Xenotransplantation. 2003. 22 figs., IX, 254 pp. ISBN 3-540-00210-3

Vol. 279: **Thomas, George; Sabatini, David; Hall, Michael N. (Eds.):** TOR. 2004. 49 figs., X, 364 pp. ISBN 3-540-00534X

Vol. 280: **Heber-Katz, Ellen (Ed.):** Regeneration: Stem Cells and Beyond. 2004. 42 figs., XII, 194 pp. ISBN 3-540-02238-4

Vol. 281: **Young, John A. T. (Ed.):** Cellular Factors Involved in Early Steps of Retroviral Replication. 2003. 21 figs., IX, 240 pp. ISBN 3-540-00844-6

Vol. 282: **Stenmark, Harald (Ed.):** Phosphoinositides in Subcellular Targeting and Enzyme Activation. 2003. 20 figs., X, 210 pp. ISBN 3-540-00950-7

Vol. 283: **Kawaoka, Yoshihiro (Ed.):** Biology of Negative Strand RNA Viruses: The Power of Reverse Genetics. 2004. 24 figs., IX, 350 pp. ISBN 3-540-40661-1

Vol. 284: **Harris, David (Ed.):** Mad Cow Disease and Related Spongiform Encephalopathies. 2004. 34 figs., IX, 219 pp. ISBN 3-540-20107-6

Vol. 285: **Marsh, Mark (Ed.):** Membrane Trafficking in Viral Replication. 2004. 19 figs., IX, 259 pp. ISBN 3-540-21430-5

Vol. 286: **Madshus, Inger H. (Ed.):** Signalling from Internalized Growth Factor Receptors. 2004. 19 figs., IX, 187 pp. ISBN 3-540-21038-5

Vol. 287: **Enjuanes, Luis (Ed.):** Coronavirus Replication and Reverse Genetics. 2005. 49 figs., XI, 257 pp. ISBN 3-540-21494-1

Vol. 288: **Mahy, Brain W. J. (Ed.):** Foot-and-Mouth-Disease Virus. 2005. 16 figs., IX, 178 pp. ISBN 3-540-22419X

Vol. 289: **Griffin, Diane E. (Ed.):** Role of Apoptosis in Infection. 2005. 40 figs., IX, 294 pp. ISBN 3-540-23006-8

Vol. 290: **Singh, Harinder; Grosschedl, Rudolf (Eds.):** Molecular Analysis of B Lymphocyte Development and Activation. 2005. 28 figs., XI, 255 pp. ISBN 3-540-23090-4

Vol. 291: **Boquet, Patrice; Lemichez Emmanuel (Eds.)** Bacterial Virulence Factors and Rho GTPases. 2005. 28 figs., IX, 196 pp. ISBN 3-540-23865-4

Vol. 292: **Fu, Zhen F (Ed.):** The World of Rhabdoviruses. 2005. 27 figs., X, 210 pp. ISBN 3-540-24011-X

Vol. 293: **Kyewski, Bruno; Suri-Payer, Elisabeth (Eds.):** CD4+CD25+ Regulatory T Cells: Origin, Function and Therapeutic Potential. 2005. 22 figs., XII, 332 pp. ISBN 3-540-24444-1

Vol. 294: **Caligaris-Cappio, Federico, Dalla Favera, Ricardo (Eds.):** Chronic Lymphocytic Leukemia. 2005. 25 figs., VIII, 187 pp. ISBN 3-540-25279-7

Vol. 295: **Sullivan, David J.; Krishna Sanjeew (Eds.):** Malaria: Drugs, Disease and Post-genomic Biology. 2005. 40 figs., XI, 446 pp. ISBN 3-540-25363-7